Health Promotion Practice

Understanding Public Health

Series editors: Nick Black and Rosalind Raine, London School of Hygiene & Tropical Medicine

Throughout the world, recognition of the importance of public health to sustainable, safe and healthy societies is growing. The achievements of public health in nineteenth-century Europe were for much of the twentieth century overshadowed by advances in personal care, in particular in hospital care. Now, with the dawning of a new century, there is increasing understanding of the inevitable limits of individual health care and of the need to complement such services with effective public health strategies. Major improvements in people's health will come from controlling communicable diseases, eradicating environmental hazards, improving people's diets and enhancing the availability and quality of effective health care. To achieve this, every country needs a cadre of knowledgeable public health practitioners with social, political and organizational skills to lead and bring about changes at international, national and local levels.

This is one of a series of 20 books that provides a foundation for those wishing to join in and contribute to the twenty-first-century regeneration of public health, helping to put the concerns and perspectives of public health at the heart of policy-making and service provision. While each book stands alone, together they provide a comprehensive account of the three main aims of public health: protecting the public from environmental hazards, improving the health of the public and ensuring high quality health services are available to all. Some of the books focus on methods, others on key topics. They have been written by staff at the London School of Hygiene & Tropical Medicine with considerable experience of teaching public health to students from low, middle and high income countries. Much of the material has been developed and tested with postgraduate students both in face-to-face teaching and through distance learning.

The books are designed for self-directed learning. Each chapter has explicit learning objectives, key terms are highlighted and the text contains many activities to enable the reader to test their own understanding of the ideas and material covered. Written in a clear and accessible style, the series will be essential reading for students taking postgraduate courses in public health and will also be of interest to public health practitioners and policy-makers.

Titles in the series

Analytical models for decision making: Colin Sanderson and Reinhold Gruen
Controlling communicable disease: Norman Noah
Economic analysis for management and policy: Stephen Jan, Lilani Kumaranayake, Jenny Roberts, Kara Hanson and Kate Archibald
Economic evaluation: Julia Fox-Rushby and John Cairns (eds)
Environmental epidemiology: Paul Wilkinson
Environment, health and sustainable development: Megan Landon
Environmental health policy: David Ball (ed)
Financial management in health services: Reinhold Gruen and Anne Howarth
Global change and health: Kelley Lee and Jeff Collin (eds)
Health care evaluation: Sarah Smith, Don Sinclair, Rosalind Raine and Barnaby Reeves
Health promotion practice: Wendy Macdowall, Chris Bonell and Maggie Davies (eds)
Health promotion theory: Maggie Davies and Wendy Macdowall (eds)
Introduction to epidemiology: Lucianne Bailey, Katerina Vardulaki, Julia Langham and Daniel Chandramohan
Introduction to health economics: David Wonderling, Reinhold Gruen and Nick Black
Issues in public health: Joceline Pomerleau and Martin McKee (eds)
Making health policy: Kent Buse, Nicholas Mays and Gill Walt
Managing health services: Nick Goodwin, Reinhold Gruen and Valerie Iles
Medical anthropology: Robert Pool and Wenzel Geissler
Principles of social research: Judith Green and John Browne (eds)
Understanding health services: Nick Black and Reinhold Gruen

Health Promotion Practice

Edited by Wendy Macdowall, Chris Bonell
and Maggie Davies

JET LIBRARY

Open University Press

Open University Press
McGraw-Hill Education
McGraw-Hill House
Shoppenhangers Road
Maidenhead
Berkshire
England
SL6 2QL

email: enquiries@openup.co.uk
world wide web: www.openup.co.uk

and Two Penn Plaza, New York, NY 10121-2289, USA

First published 2006

Reprinted 2007 (twice)

A catalogue record of this book is available from the British Library

ISBN-10: 0 335 218407 (pb)
ISBN-13: 978 0 335 218400 (pb)

Library of Congress Cataloging-in-Publication Data
CIP data has been applied for

Typeset by RefineCatch Limited, Bungay, Suffolk
Printed in Great Britain by Bell & Bain Ltd., Glasgow

Contents

Acknowledgements

Health Promotion International by Johnson, A. et al. Copyright 2001 by Oxford University Press – Journals. Reproduced with permission of Oxford University Press – Journals in the format textbook via Copyright Clearance Center. Table 12.2

Department of Health (2005) National Healthy Schools Status – A Guide for Schools. © Crown copyright. Chapter 12 text extracts

Reproduced with permission from Harden et al (2001) *Peer-delivered health promotion for young people: a systematic review of different study designs*, Copyright © Health Education Journal, 2001, by permission of Sage Publications Ltd. Figure 3.5

'The Marketing Plan'. Source: Adapted from Hastings and Elliot (1993) reproduced in Road Transport and Intermodal Linkages Research Programme Marketing of Traffic Safety, © OECD 1993 Figure 10.3

Hickson, F et al (2003) Making it Count, 3rd edition. Table 1.1

Jackson, N & Waters, E. for the Guidelines for Systematic Reviews of Health Promotion and Public Health Interventions Task Force (2005a) *Guidelines for systematic reviews of health promotion and public health interventions, Version 1.2*. Melbourne, Australia. Deakin University, April 2005. Also Table 3.1

McKnight, J. (1996) *The Careless Society: community and its counterfeits* Copyright © Basic Books. Figures 2.1 & 2.2

Oliver, S & Peersman G. (2001) *Using Research for Effective Health Promotion*. © Copyright 2001, Open University Press. Reproduced with the kind permission of the Open University Press / McGraw-Hill Publishing Company. Table 3.1, Figure 3.1, Figure 3.3 & Figure 3.4

Adapted from Health Education Research by Stead, M., Hastings, G. & Eadie, D. Copyright 2002 by Oxford University Press – Journals. Reproduced with permission of Oxford University Press – Journals in the format Textbook via Copyright Clearance Center. Figure 9.2

Wellings, K and MacDowall W. 'Evaluating mass media approaches' in Coombes, Y & Thorogood, M (eds), *Evaluation of Health Promotion* (2004). Copyright Oxford University Press. Chapter 8 text

Health Promotion International by Whitelaw, S. et al, Copyright 2001 by Oxford University Press - Journals. Reproduced with permission of Oxford University Press - Journals in the format Textbook by Copyright Clearance Center. Table 12.1

Overview of the book

Introduction

Health promotion is generally regarded as aiming to increase control over the multi-levelled and complex determinants of health and illness using social interventions. To do this, health promotion should address individual attributes and behaviours, the social norms that influence these, and the wider distribution of rights, responsibilities and resources within societies that are the 'upstream' influences on these factors. The development of interventions is facilitated by: the use of theory; understanding the determinants of health and illness; assessing the needs of populations; understanding the approaches to promoting health and their strengths and weaknesses; programme planning; and rigorous evaluation. The focus of this book is on the last four of these elements. The book builds on another book in the Understanding Public Health series, called *Health Promotion Theory*, in which the first two 'ingredients' are explored.

Structure of the book

Each chapter follows the same format. A brief overview tells you about the contents, followed by learning objectives and the key terms you will encounter. There are activities which are designed to encourage you to think about an issue, or to test your knowledge and understanding. Each activity is followed by feedback to enable you to check on your own understanding. The book is arranged in three sections which take you through the groundwork in developing interventions, the methods and approaches which form the interventions, and delivery and reflection on practice.

The groundwork

The focus of Chapter 1 is on developing a programmatic approach to health promotion. It is argued that health promoters must be clear what they are aiming to achieve – i.e. what 'needs' they will be addressing. In Chapter 2 you will learn about needs assessment. The chapter considers how 'health states' and 'needs for interventions' can be measured including use of routine and ad hoc data. Using empirical research to inform health promotion is a complex matter. In Chapter 3 you will learn about some approaches to searching and appraising critically research evidence that can provide health promotion planners with some of the information they require.

Choosing approaches and methods

In this section you will be introduced to different methods and approaches commonly used in health promotion to address individual, community and societal determinants of health and illness. The groundwork should have led you to the conclusion that there isn't a simple divide between effective and ineffective methods. Instead different methods will be effective at achieving different aims with different groups in different settings. A health promotion programme which is designed to address the multiple determinants of a public health problem is likely to consist of a number of interventions. So although necessarily arranged in discrete chapters, you should consider these methods and approaches as potentially complementary rather than as competitors.

Individual level

While it may be the case that health promotion programmes have focused on individual determinants to the neglect of addressing social influences, there is still an important role for health promotion in enabling individuals to appraise and modify their own health behaviour. Chapter 4 explores such individual-focused approaches and methods. In Chapter 5 you will learn about an approach for communicating with people during face-to-face interventions called motivational interviewing. A central tenet of this approach is the exploration and resolution of ambivalence about behaviour change. The motivational interviewer's task is to facilitate expression of both sides of the ambivalence and guide the client towards an acceptable resolution that increases the probability of positive change.

Group or community level

Arts-based activities are now widely recognized as useful tools of public health across the world. In Chapter 6 you will be introduced to use of theatre in health promotion and the range of theatre techniques available to support public health and development programmes. Chapter 7 examines what is meant by peer education and outlines some of the theories associated with this approach. Peer education has become popular with practitioners and has incorporated a diverse range of approaches and addressed a wide variety of health issues.

The mass media

The mass media can play a significant role in public health; both good and bad. In Chapters 8 and 9, you will learn about two methods that utilize the mass media. The first of these is mass media campaigns. It is argued that where mass media interventions work, it is more likely to be because they activate a complex process of change in social norms rather than because they directly change individual behaviour. In Chapter 9 you will learn about media advocacy as an approach to public health policy change, and compare and contrast it with other techniques such as lobbying, advocacy and public relations.

Approaches

These chapters bring together different approaches that inform the development of health promotion interventions. They are not 'methods' *per se* but can be considered as different philosophical standpoints which place either the consumer, the community or the setting at the core. The first of these, which you will learn about in Chapter 10, is social marketing. Social marketing takes ideas and techniques that are used in the commercial sector to influence *consumer* behaviour and applies them to *health* behaviour.

Chapter 11 looks at community development, an approach that seeks to empower communities to recognize, confront and develop solutions to the issues that affect them. The philosphy here is that the community itself has the greatest understanding of the issues that it faces and when 'empowered' knows the best ways to address these issues.

Chapter 12 introduces 'settings-based health promotion', a concept developed and supported by the World Health Organization (WHO) since its first mention in the Ottawa Charter in 1986. It embodies a holistic (whole system) philosophy. The chapter provides examples of programmes that have attempted to translate the rhetoric into practical action and contrasts 'projectism' with the structural and organizational changes necessary for hospitals, schools and other settings to become truly health promoting.

Influencing policy

Research has repeatedly demonstrated the importance of social conditions in influencing the health of individuals and populations. Chapter 13 considers how government policies – as major drivers of social conditions – may contribute to health, and gives examples of how they may reduce, and sometimes increase, health inequalities. It also considers the role of health impact assessment in informing health public policies, and discusses how better evidence on healthy public policy can be obtained.

Delivery and reflection

Having considered how to devise health promotion programmes and the strengths and weakness of different methods for achieving specific aims and objectives, the next stage is delivery. Successful delivery of health promotion requires sound project management from planning through implementation to completion. In Chapter 14 you will explore the different tasks involved in project management and how to undertake these tasks. Chapter 15 considers evaluation and argues that rigorous evaluation of outcomes and of processes is important but that before evaluation designs and methods are chosen, the evaluation questions must be specified. The chapter goes on to discuss the roles of different sorts of data and different study designs. The final chapter, Chapter 16, looks at the issue of intervention transfer and in particular generalizability and scale-up of health promotion interventions.

Acknowledgments

The book is based on two teaching units at the London School of Hygiene & Tropical Medicine, namely Principles and Practice of Health Promotion and the Health Promotion Integrating Unit. These courses have evolved over several years under the influence of Yolande Combes, Nicki Thorogood, Spencer Haggard, Adam Biran and many others. The editors are grateful to Jenny Douglas, Senior Lecturer in Health Promotion at the Open University, for comments on the first draft, Nick Black, Professor of Health Services Research for editorial input and Rachael Parker and Avril Porter for administrative support.

Authors

Wendy Macdowall is a Lecturer in Health Promotion, *Chris Bonell* is a Senior Lecturer in Social Science & Epidemiology, *James Hargreaves* is a Lecturer in Epidemiology and *Kaye Wellings* is Professor of Sexual and Reproductive Health, London School of Hygiene & Tropical Medicine; *Maggie Davies* is Principal Advisor in International Health Development at the Department of Health; *Ford Hickson* is a Senior Research Fellow at Sigma Research, University of Portsmouth; *Antony Morgan* is Associate Director of Research at the National Institute for Health and Clinical Excellence; *Ginny Brunton, Helen Burchett, Rebecca Rees* and *Vicki Strange* are Research Officers and *Meg Wiggins* is Assistant Director, Social Science Research Unit, Institute of Education; *Oliver Davidson* is an Associate Professor in the Department of Psychological Medicine, Dunedin School of Medicine, University of Otago; *Melvyn Hillsdon* is Senior Lecturer in Exercise and Health Science at the University of Bristol; *Roy Head* is Director of Development Media International; *Martine Stead* is Deputy Director and *Gerard Hastings* is Professor of Social Marketing and Director of the Institute of Social Marketing, University of Stirling; *Rhian Twine* is the coordinator of the LinC office of the Wits/MRC Agincourt Health and Population Unit, University of the Witwatersrand; *Mark Petticrew* is Associate Director and *Matt Egan* is a Research Associate at the MRC Social and Public Health Sciences Unit, University of Glasgow; *Viv Speller* is a freelance public health consultant; and *Fiona Sawney* and *Liza Cragg* are freelance consultants.

SECTION 1

The groundwork

Developing a programmatic approach to health promotion

Overview

The focus of this chapter is on developing a programmatic approach to health promotion. You will consider what is required for something to be called an intervention rather than just an activity and will be introduced to a number of intervention qualities that can be investigated. Examples from HIV infection in Britain, in particular a bio-psycho-social model of HIV incidence that is currently used to plan HIV prevention programmes will be used throughout the chapter. This will allow you to consider the larger question of what needs to change in order to develop a programmatic approach to increasing health in a population.

Learning objectives

After reading this chapter, you will be better able to:

- understand what is meant by a health promotion need
- distinguish health-related behaviours from health-related needs
- describe the way in which health promotion attempts to influence people to change their behaviour
- identify a range of intervention targets and needs that may be addressed to improved the health of a population
- understand what are meant by a health promotion intervention and health promotion programme
- plan health promotion programmes that address multiple needs

Key terms

Aim An expanded and refined version of a goal that sets out the means by which the end point, in general terms, is to be attained.

Health-related behaviour Things people do that affect their health (e.g. sexual activity that involves exposure to infections).

Health-related needs Attributes people need to have to be able to control their health-related behaviour: knowledge and awareness; access to resources; interpersonal skills and physical motor skills; and bodily autonomy.

Intervention A purposeful activity using finite resources that occurs in a specific place with the aim of changing something specific for a specific person or group of people.

Objective Concrete and specific elaboration of an aim.

Programme A collection of interventions that share an overall health-related goal.

Setting (site) The place or location in which intervention activities occur.

Introduction

States of health and disease are influenced by various behaviours. For example, eating a balanced diet or taking antibiotics reduce the risk of some diseases and engaging in unprotected sex or breathing asbestos increase the risk of others. In turn, whether individuals engage in such behaviours is influenced by whether people possess various things required to have maximum control over their behaviour – i.e. whether various 'needs' are met or not. For example, whether someone eats a balanced diet or not may be influenced by whether their need for accurate information about nutrition has been met or not; whether someone engages in unprotected sex or not may be in part influenced by whether their need for developing interpersonal sexual negotiation skills has been met or not. We can identify needs by asking the individuals themselves (i.e. 'expressed' need) or by 'experts' identifying on the basis of logic or research what someone might need (i.e. 'normative' need). Most complex behaviours are associated with a number of different needs (e.g. knowledge, interpersonal skills, access to resources). In addition, different people may require different interventions to meet the same need. For example, knowledge may be gained by some through a leaflet while others may require a face-to-face conversation.

The extent to which individuals' identified health needs are met is dictated by the actions of policy-makers, education, health and social services and communities. There is not always a sharp distinction between these constituencies but the distinction is worth retaining to illustrate the diversity of actors and actions for health. Policy-makers include central and local governments and strategic decision-makers in organizations, and it is policy-makers – rather than the people delivering the services – who usually determine which and how services are delivered. Further, everyone is a member of one or more 'community' and people get many of their health-related needs met by the people they live with and are around on a daily basis, making them important vectors for health too.

Each of the three constituencies (policy-makers, services and communities) influences the health of others as a result either of their planned or unplanned intervention or as a result of their not intervening. These constituencies' activities are themselves dictated by the extent to which their own 'needs for action' are met. 'Need for action' here refers to the things that these people need to have, such as information, institutional capacity and favourable attitudes, in order to intervene in a useful manner. An overall goal to improve the health of a population may involve interventions targeted at the needs of these three constituencies to act in the interests of the population, as well as (or even instead of) interventions targeted at the population itself. It follows that no one type of intervention will be able to meet all needs associated with a health issue for all people. Consequently, a collection of interventions is usually needed to address any health issue. A collection of interventions is called a programme.

The relationships between health outcomes, behaviours and needs are complex and often poorly understood. Most interventions are able to impact on a number of needs, most needs are associated with a number of behaviours and most behaviours have impacts on more than one health outcome. Conversely, how frequently a disease occurs in a population (its *incidence*) is related to many biological, psychological and social factors. Not all of these are amenable to change through medicine or health promotion and therefore not all can be thought of in terms of 'need'. Many diseases have multiple risk behaviours associated with them and the incidence of each risk behaviour in a population influences the incidence of several health outcomes. For example, the frequency of unprotected sexual intercourse between people with and without HIV infection will influence how frequently HIV is transmitted (only a proportion of these events will result in transmission). How frequently this occurs will be influenced by rate of partner change in the population and the overall frequency of unprotected intercourse. These two factors will also influence the incidence of other sexually transmitted infections, as well as pregnancies. So the same population behaviours have multiple health impacts.

It follows then that any unmet health need is likely to impact on several health-related behaviours. For example, lack of assertiveness makes safer sexual negotiation more difficult and reduces ability to resist peer pressure around smoking and drinking, as well as disadvantaging people in the health market-place. This is part of the explanation for why different types of ill health cluster in the same people.

We can't guarantee that by meeting what have been identified as needs will lead to changes in behaviour that promote health. In some cases, despite addressing a number of important health-related needs, others remain unidentified and therefore unmet. For example, health promoters might fail to identify the need to be able to access healthy foods as an influence on whether someone eats a balanced diet. Therefore, the behaviour changes that health promoters hoped to see don't materialize. Furthermore, people may simply decide that they do not want to change behaviour, despite their 'needs' being met.

It is important to recognize that people have different views as to what is acceptable to do to people to influence their behaviour. Some see the acceptable limit of health promotion as enabling individuals to have maximum control over the determinants of their health. In other words, health promotion should restrict itself to meeting people's needs as defined earlier. Others judge it acceptable to go beyond this to influence behaviour through other means as well. Such people might see health promotion activities as including empowering people to make healthy choices where they want to, but in some cases might also see it as legitimate to direct people's actions in non-empowering ways. They might for example see it as legitimate to pressurize people into eating balanced diets by increasing taxes on fatty foods or by curbing the availability of fast-food restaurants via planning regulations. Some might even see it as acceptable to outlaw certain kinds of sexual practice, scare people, misinform them or interfere with their civil liberties in other ways such as curbing their freedom of movement. It is important to recognize that both approaches share the same behavioural goal for the population (e.g. increased fruit and vegetable intake or fewer sexual HIV exposures); they differ in what sorts of changes they are willing to bring about in order to ensure those behaviours occur.

What one views as acceptable means of influence will determine how one evaluates the success of health promotion interventions. If the approach to behaviour change is solely in terms of empowering people to make their own choices, one would evaluate health promotion mostly in terms of the extent to which it meets identified needs as well as the behaviour it is intended to influence. If one views health promotion as aiming to influence behaviours by any means necessary, including empowering and in some cases directive ones, one would primarily focus on changes in behaviour or health status, although one might also want to examine other factors such as whether needs have been met in order to understand *how* interventions may have worked.

Why describe interventions?

In health promotion planning and delivery there are three common reasons why we might want to describe interventions. The first is to buy and sell them. Agencies wishing to undertake interventions usually have to raise funds to do so, and a key task here is conveying the essence of the intervention to potential funders. Conversely, health commissioners often wish to bring particular interventions into being and must issue a tender for them, in the process describing the intervention they wish to purchase.

The second common reason for describing interventions is in order to evaluate them (evaluation is covered in Chapter 15). Although it is possible to make some judgements of undescribed activities it is not possible to say anything about the key intervention performance parameters without an intervention description. So for example, unless we say something about the intended target for an intervention, we are unable to address questions of equity of access; if we know nothing about the resources required for an intervention (or how many people got it), we cannot talk about its unit costs. Most importantly though, if we have no aim for an intervention we cannot say whether or not it is effective.

The third reason for describing interventions is to replicate them. An intervention description then can also be a record of what to do if you want to implement it. Interventions that do what we want them to do, for the people we intend them to do it for, are valuable. An intervention that met the needs of some people in one place may well meet another group of people's needs somewhere else (see Chapter 16 for some of the issues related to intervention transfer). Without an intervention description it can be difficult or impossible for someone else (or even ourselves) to run it again.

These are not all the uses of intervention descriptions, but buying and selling, evaluating and replicating interventions would all be impossible in their absence. The amount of detail an intervention description contains will depend on what it is being used for. For example, a description of an intervention used to raise funds need not contain as much detail as one intended to allow someone else to replicate the intervention in the future. The easiest way of avoiding explicit failure is to decline to specify what success would look like. Intervention evaluations are often over-optimistic about the performance of interventions because the intervention is so poorly specified as to make it difficult to fail. For example, many interventions state what will happen (the objectives) but not what is hoped to change (the aim). Simply having done the intervention is therefore judged a success. Similarly, stating the target group to be the people using the setting (e.g. schoolchildren, bar users etc.) means the intervention cannot fail in encountering its target group.

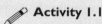

Activity 1.1

Read the description of an intervention in a journal article reporting an evaluation. Is the intervention described in enough detail for you to replicate it in precisely the same way? Does the report include the cost of the intervention? What other information is missing?

Feedback

Few journal articles describe interventions in enough detail to replicate them and fewer still include the monetary cost of the intervention.

What constitutes an intervention description?

Interventions are purposeful and planned actions intended to contribute to a reduction in unmet health-related need (and hence a reduction in illness-related behaviour or an increase in health-related behaviours). As you have learnt, they include actions directed towards, for example, government ministers, newspaper editors and service commissioners as well as actions directed at the population of concern.

Without a *purpose* and a *plan*, an activity should not be considered an intervention. The purpose for a health-related intervention is to address the requirements for action, or needs, in a specific person or group of people. The needs are defined by the health- or illness-related behaviour they are attached to (needs assessment is considered in Chapter 2). The plan consists of a number of activities that take place in a specific location, the site of the intervention. In order to complete an intervention description, we should say something about the resources required to do the intervention. So there are five essential elements to all intervention descriptions: aim, setting, target, objectives and resources.

Intervention aims

As discussed above, different people approach influencing behaviours in different ways. Some approach behaviour change through reducing the needs of the target of the intervention. Others may seek to influence behaviour via empowering people to make their own decisions (e.g. educating people about a healthy diet) and sometimes by using more directive means (e.g. taxing foods with high fat content). Which, if either, approach is effective will vary depending on the behaviour under consideration. If we take the view that empowered populations act in their own interests and make healthier decisions than disempowered populations, interventions should aim to influence needs. In other words, the success of a specified intervention is defined by its impact on needs. See Chapter 16 for an alternative argument that evaluations should focus both on such needs and on other outcomes such as changes in health behaviours and health states.

The remainder of this chapter argues for evaluation to focus primarily on outcomes concerned with reductions in need. Needs in this case are defined as the requirements for control over health-related behaviours. For example, in the case of HIV risk behaviours, HIV prevention needs may include physical autonomy (freedom from assault and rape), assertiveness skills, ability to negotiate safer sex (interpersonal skills), ability to establish one's own HIV status (i.e. access to HIV testing), access to condoms and the knowledge and ability to use them properly, knowledge and awareness of HIV and its prevention etc. What we judge the needs related to a behaviour to be are related to our theories about why people do what they do, our judgements about what can be changed by interventions and our ethical position about what interventions should do.

One way to elucidate the aims of an intervention is to answer the question *In what way is the target group different after the intervention objectives have occurred?* It is important not to fall back on the behaviours of the target group here. Since different people may do the same thing for different reasons, and since the same people may do different things for the same reason, any behaviour may be associated with a wide range of needs. Interventions do not change people's behaviours. Interventions (sometimes) change people, and people change their behaviours.

Intervention settings and sites

Settings specify how the people the intervention is intended to change encounter the intervention activities. All intervention objectives must take place somewhere and the place they occur in is a key determinant of both their feasibility and the profile of the people who encounter them. Although no specific activities can be done everywhere, there are few places in which no health promotion activities can be done. This means the potential range of settings for health promotion interventions is enormous. Interventions intended to reduce health-related needs can be carried out in: the media (press, radio, television); the street; socializing business (pubs, clubs, restaurants); schools; community and religious centres (including churches, mosques, synagogues); service centres (clinics, organizational bases); care-homes; prisons; personal homes.

In addition, interventions targeted at the needs for action of, for example, policy-makers and service providers can occur through professional networks. In these cases, the potential targets may hear about the intervention through being contacted directly.

Many of these settings are places where people are present for some reason other than health promotion activities. Activities in these settings do not usually require a front-end (the people are already there). Interventions occurring in places where people have to attend (i.e. where the intervened on come to the intervenor) usually require an additional intervention (recruitment) in a place where people are already (including, e.g., reading press magazines and newspapers). Where these front-end interventions occur will dictate who attends.

Intervention targets

Target groups are defined to maximize the impact of the intervention through trying to ensure the people who encounter the intervention are those in most need of it. Descriptions of target groups are therefore in some ways surrogate markers for a combination of the health concern at issue or the specific unmet needs the intervention addresses. However, interventions are not always targeted at those most likely to suffer from an illness or most likely to have a need unmet. Very few interventions can aspire to serve people equally irrespective of where they live in a country (there are, e.g., few 'national' interventions). The interests of the funder of the intervention and the values of the intervenor both mediate between need and target group.

The specified target should be as comprehensive as possible and aspects of the target group not mentioned should be assumed to be equally served by the intervention. So, for example, 'young people' does not mean 'young heterosexual people' unless it explicitly says so. An intervention whose target is simply 'young people' should be expected to be of equal benefit to gay/lesbian and heterosexual young people, young people from ethnic minorities as well as the ethnic majority, disabled young people as well as able-bodied young people, and so on. It should also be expected equally to benefit young men as well as young women, unless specified otherwise.

The profile of people whose needs are intended to change as a result of intervention activities can include consideration of gender, age, ethnicity, sexuality, disability, class/occupation/education, area of residence, as well as other characteristics. If the intervention is targeted at service providers or policy-makers, the intervention description should be as precise as possible about who these people are. In this case, the potential target audience is usually much smaller than the potential target audience among the general public.

✎ Activity 1.2

Study the specified target group for an intervention (either a health promoter's description or in an evaluation report). Does it include information about where the intended target group live, their sex, age, ethnicity, sexuality, disability, occupation or education? What other characteristics are mentioned (exclude those based on where the intervention occurs or on what the aim of the intervention is)? Considering these seven characteristics (residence, sex, age, ethnicity, sexuality, disability, education/occupation level), which sub-groups do you think are more likely to encounter the intervention than others?

Feedback

The term 'general population' is often used to ignore desirable and undesirable biases in interventions. There is no health issue that is equally distributed across all characteristics of the population. No intervention is encountered by all members of its target group and all interventions have target group biases. For example, mass media interventions are disproportionately seen by some sections of their target group more than others, places on skills courses are taken more frequently by some groups. The target group for an intervention should specify, where relevant, the desirable biases in who gets the intervention more than others. For example, is the intervention intended to be encountered equally by those with no educational qualifications as by those with university education? If not, which group is intended to be served more than others?

Intervention objectives

Generally, aims are where you want to be and objectives are what you do to get there. What constitutes an objective depends on where an aim is pitched. For example, if our aim is reducing new sexually-acquired HIV infections, our objectives could be to reduce sexual HIV exposures and the biological factors that facilitate transmission (e.g. concurrent STIs, body fluid transfer, increasing post-exposure prophylaxis etc.). Subsequently, if our aim is reducing sexual HIV exposure, our objectives could be to increase knowledge, awareness, skills, access to condoms, etc. Then if our aim is to increase knowledge, our objectives could be to write, design, produce and distribute an information leaflet.

At the most immediate and basic level then, objectives are the things that you do that constitute the intervention. This is the first level at which objectives can be specified and it is what is meant when we refer to intervention objectives. Objectives include the sequence of events that occur as well as the methods and approaches being used. The different methods and approaches commonly used in health promotion to address individual, community and societal determinants of health and illness are covered in Chapters 4 to 13. There is not a simple divide between 'effective' and 'ineffective' methods; rather, different methods are more or less effective at achieving different aims with different groups in different settings.

Note that the objectives include what the people being intervened on do as well as what the intervenor does. An intervention cannot be said to have occurred if a leaflet is put in a rack but no one ever takes it and reads it. It is the act of reading the leaflet that completes the objectives of the intervention.

Small media such as leaflets and postcards require a distribution mechanism to get them into people's hands. So, for example, 'a leaflet' is not in itself an intervention. Similarly, some objectives are incomplete without a 'front-end'. Recruitment is often half of an intervention and should be included in the description of the activities.

Intervention resources

A description of an intervention should say something about the resources required to carry it out. While this can be expressed as money, there may also be some resources required to do the intervention that cannot be purchased by the health promoter. So for example, an outreach session in a gay bar requires: trained workers, resources to distribute (leaflets, condoms etc.) and a gay bar in which to carry out the work. The objectives could include: arrangement with bar owner/manager to visit and work the site; attending the site; approaching and engaging clients; talking and listening to establish and address unmet needs; and distributing leaflets and condoms.

Who is responsible for the health needs of a population?

There are numerous health issues unequally distributed between and within countries. The size and nature of national responses to health issues varies, both over time and across populations. Whether a health issue is responded to is often related to who is being affected by it. Health issues which are limited to unpopular or marginalized populations (such as HIV, tuberculosis or sickle-cell anaemia) are less likely to garner public and political support for action than are those which affect either the 'general population' or politically safe populations such as children. This means that if we wish to impact on health issues affecting 'unpopular' populations we must also address the political context in which the health promotion is carried out (or not). To a large extent though this is also true for all health issues.

The success of national responses to health issues rests on the commitment of diverse constituencies of people and organizations. As such, they demand a multi-level approach to realize their goals. Moreover, there exists no one agency or institution with overall responsibility for any single health issue nor any single group of organizations commanding sufficient expertise, resources and respect to ensure that an issue is comprehensively tackled. All health issues have a number of agencies and organizations working on them, and the extent to which each of them succeeds depends on its relationship and complementarity to all the others. Hence collective success depends crucially on the degree and success of collaboration.

Policy-makers and commissioners, service providers and the community share the need for a collective, coherent and coordinated response to health issues. With an increase in the numbers and types of players engaged in the response to health issues there is a concomitant need for partnerships, referrals and exchange of learning. These needs also require addressing and are appropriate aims for health promotion interventions.

A typology of preventative action

This chapter has identified that some view acceptable health promotion as empowering people in order to influence their health-related behaviours while others believe that in some cases directive means can also be used. As many stakeholders are involved in addressing or undermining needs, health promotion actions involve many groups of people other than the people whose health-related behaviour we are concerned with.

Hence health promotion is affected by all policy areas, services and the common conduct of most of the population. Many of these actions make health-related needs *worse*, especially with regards to the needs of socially unpopular groups, such as, for example, immigrants, gay men or prisoners. The social epidemics of homophobia and discrimination associated with HIV, for example, have fed the viral epidemic since its inception. Much HIV prevention activity has been spent addressing these obstacles precisely among those people who could have been contributing to a reduction in HIV incidence. Health promotion programmes often seek to increase health-promoting activity in others, as well as directly reducing the unmet health needs in the population of concern.

Any action that contributes towards meeting health-related needs for any target groups can be recognized as a valid health promotion activity. This means it is possible to have interventions that make a significant contribution to increasing health without directly addressing health-related behaviours. From the preceding it should be clear that a health promotion action can be carried out by:

- community members;
- policy-makers, researchers and resource allocators;
- education, health and social services personnel.

It should also be clear that a health promotion action can be targeted at:

- the illness- and health-related needs of people whose behaviours we are concerned about;
- the needs of community members (knowledge, skills, resources) to carry out health promotion actions (e.g. advocating health-related behaviours in peers, cooking balanced meals for families);
- policy-makers, researchers and resource allocators' needs (knowledge, skills, resources) for health promotion actions;
- education, health and social services personnel's needs (knowledge, skills, resources) for health promotion actions.

Table 1.1 outlines the range of elements of a response to a health issue. The specific examples relate to the HIV epidemic among homosexually active men, but the categories of intervention are applicable to all health issues. The typology gives us 12 different types of intervention in three groups of four. Usually health promoters will only consider the interventions they themselves do, but they also have a major role in encouraging interventions by others.

Table 1.1 A typology of health promotion action: building a programme

Actors	Target of action	Examples of interventions in a national HIV prevention programme
Policy-makers, resource allocators & researchers	Policy-makers', researchers' & resource allocators' action needs	National evidence base programme
		Public funds
	Service providers' action needs	National and local prevention strategies/plans
		Development of HIV vaccines and microbicides
	Community action needs	Leadership against stigma and discrimination
	Population of concern's health-related needs	Social equality & justice legislation
Education, health and social service providers	Policy-makers', researchers' & resource allocators' action needs	Professional associations and representation in policy-making, research & resource allocation
	Service providers' action needs	Training & professional development
		National & local collaborative planning fora
	Community action needs	Community development
	Population of concern's health-related needs	Equitable generic education, health & social services • HIV education & counselling • Condoms & lubricant distribution • Access to HIV & STI diagnosis & treatment
Community members	Policy-makers', researchers' & resource allocators' action needs	Political action and lobbying
	Service providers' action needs	Gay public involvement in service planning
	Community action needs	Voluntary associations and community mobilization
	Population of concern's health-related needs	Peer education

Source: Hickson *et al.* (2003)

Activity 1.3

Choose a major health issue in your country. Imagine you work in a non-governmental organization (NGO) dedicated to that issue. Using the typology above, identify one potential intervention for each cell of the typology. Write a few words on the aim, setting, target, objectives and resources for each intervention. Assuming you have a limited budget, which interventions would you prioritize?

 Feedback

The most appropriate programme for a health issue will depend on the current awareness and response to the issue among community members, services and policy-makers. It will also depend on the values and approach of your NGO.

Where to start planning an intervention

All interventions have the dimensions Aim, Setting, Target, Objectives and Resources. The mnemonic ASTOR is a way of remembering these five dimensions. An intervention can however be planned starting at any of the five dimensions but once one or two of the dimensions are specified, the others become limited in what they can be (the choices become narrower).

Start with an aim/need
  Who has the aim/need poorly met?
    Where can they be encountered?
      What activities that reduce the need can be done there?
        What resources are required?

Start with a target group
  What needs do they have unmet?
    Where can they be encountered?
      What activities that reduce the need can be done there?
        What resources are required?

Start with some resources
  Whose needs do you want to address?
    What needs/aims do they have poorly met?
      Where can they be encountered?
        What can be done there within the resources that will address unmet needs?

Start with a setting
  What activities can be done there?
    Who can be encountered there?
      What unmet needs do they have that can be addressed with feasible activities?
        What resources are required?

Start with objectives/tools
    What resources are required?
        Where can the objectives be done?
            Who can be encountered there?
                What needs that can be addressed by the available tools do the target have unmet?

Activity 1.4

Return to the health issue you chose in Activity 1.3. Using the steps above develop five interventions, one from each of the following starting points: (1) the factors associated with the behavioural aspect of your chosen health issue that are amenable to change through intervention; (2) the health issue as it affects middle-aged men (remember, they may act as advocates for others); (3) 50,000 euros to spend on the health issue; (4) an intervention that can be done in a local department store which is concerned about the issue (could be with either employees or customers); (5) an intervention employing advertisements and small group discussions. For each of the five interventions check that the objectives can be carried out in the setting and within the budget (feasibility) and that the budget is not excessive for the activities (efficiency). Also check that you have specified the target group for each intervention and that it matches the setting in which the activities will be carried out (accessibility to target group).

Feedback

Although the five interventions you have outlined will probably have different impacts on the incidence of the health issue you are concerned about, they may not all be equally available to your NGO. The existing relationships with other stakeholders, the budget available, the accessibility of the target group and the expertise of the health promoters with different tools will all limit which actions are available.

The goal in intervention planning is to develop a coherent intervention (planning is covered in greater detail in Chapter 14). That is, one whose objectives can be carried out in the setting (feasible), within the resources (affordable), are agreeable to the target group (acceptable), which can bring about change in the aim (effective) and whose target group is encountered in the setting (accessible) and do not already have the aim of the intervention met (needed).

Where we start planning an intervention from will depend on who we are, what our role is and who our collaborators are. Government policy often determines which diseases and target groups funding is available for and guides the activity of statutory bodies. The intervention portfolio of any health promotion department is influenced by the interests and expertise of the current staff team as well as the unit's history. Interventions also follow fashions and different diseases and population groups become more or less popular as do different tools and settings. However, evidence of the saliency of a disease in the local population and its distribution in different sectors of the community should always be attended to.

Summary

What is and is not a health-related need is a matter of both evidence and values. We need evidence that a behaviour is related to the heath issue we are concerned about, and we need evidence that any particular factor is indeed related to the behaviour. For example, is lung cancer related to smoking, and is smoking related to the price of tobacco, are two different hypotheses, both of which need evidence to support them before manipulating the price of tobacco can be adopted as an aim of a (policy) intervention to reduce lung cancer.

There is no set of intervention objectives that can be done anywhere, cost very little, are liked by everyone and can address all needs, for all people. Therefore no single intervention is able to tackle any one health issue, even less so the range of health needs for any single population. So for any health issue, or the health of any population, a programme of interventions is required that complement each other and work together to cover the varied needs of a population.

References

Hickson F, Nutland W, Weatherburn P, Burnell C, Keogh M, Doyle T, Watson R, Gault A (2003) *Making It Count: A collaborative planning framework to reduce the incidence of HIV infection during sex between men*, 3rd edn. London: Sigma Research (available at: www.sigmaresearch.org.uk).

Further reading

Devlin W, Keogh P, Nutland W, Weatherburn P (2003) *The Field Guide: applying Making it Count to health promotion activity with homosexually active men*. London: Terrence Higgins Trust.

Ellis S, Barnett-Page E, Morgan A, Taylor L, Walters R, Goodrich J (2003) *HIV prevention: a review of reviews assessing the effectiveness of interventions to reduce the risk of sexual transmission: evidence briefing*. London: Health Development Agency (available at: www.publichealth.nice.org.uk/page.aspx?o=502573).

Hickson F, Hartley M, Weatherburn P (2000) *London Counts: HIV prevention needs and interventions among gay and bisexual men in the sixteen London Health Authorities*. London: Sigma Research (available at: www.sigmaresearch.org.uk).

2 Needs assessment

Overview

Needs assessment in health promotion is essential in the development of appropriate policy and programmatic solutions to public health concerns. It is commonly used to review the health issues of populations, to identify and agree the priorities for action and to demonstrate the most efficient and cost-effective use of scarce resources in the public sector.

In this chapter, you will learn the importance of needs assessment, the processes involved in carrying out needs assessment, the data sources most commonly used and some of the current issues relating to this area of work.

Learning objectives

After reading this chapter, you will be better able to:

- describe the rationale for needs assessment in health promotion
- describe the main stages involved in a needs assessment study
- identify some of the major sources of information required to complete a study
- distinguish the relationship between a range of tools and techniques relevant to assessing the health priorities of local communities

Key terms

Community asset mapping An inventory of the strengths (assets) of the people who make up a community; the interconnections of these assets and how to access them.

Health equity auditing (HEA) Identifies how fairly services or other resources are distributed in relation to the health needs of different groups and areas, and the priority action to provide services.

Health impact assessment An approach to ensure that decision-making at all levels considers the potential impacts of decisions on health and health inequalities, and identifies actions that can enhance positive effects and reduce or eliminate negative effects.

Health needs assessment A systematic process of identifying priority health issues, targeting the populations with most need and taking action in the most cost-effective and efficient way.

What is a needs assessment and why do it?

Rising demands in health care, limited resources and increasing inequalities in health are some of the main drivers for needs assessment studies in European countries (WHO 2001). Wright *et al.* (1998) report that over the last 30 years health care expenditures in most developed countries have risen faster than the cost increases reported in other sectors and that medical advances and demographic changes will force costs and demands on health services to rise further. There is increasing evidence to suggest that spending more on health care will not result in significant improvements in population health. Governments are therefore increasingly looking to the potential for prevention activities to alleviate some of the burden from heath care services.

Cavanagh and Chadwick (2005) define health needs assessment as 'a systematic process of identifying priority health issues, targeting the populations with most need and taking action in the most cost effective and efficient way'. This definition encapsulates both the purpose and desired outcome of a good needs assessment study. So while the *purpose* of needs assessment is to determine health priorities and unmet health and social need the *desired outcome* should be action to address the needs identified to ensure improvements in health are made. There are a number of other reasons why needs assessment is important in health promotion as illustrated in Table 2.1.

Basic needs assessment has been the cornerstone of health promotion and public health activity for many years and has traditionally involved providing epidemiological assessments of the state of population health to help determine priorities for action. These have been conducted at the international, national and local levels. They all in some way help decision-makers choose where investments in health should be made to deliver the most health gain. In some countries, needs assessment activities are becoming a statutory requirement to ensure that scarce resources in the health sector can be maximized. For example, in England, health authorities are required by the 1990 National Health Service Act to assess the health needs of their populations and to use these assessments to set priorities to improve the health of their local population (Wright *et al.* 1998).

Table 2.1 Why is health needs assessment important for health promotion?

- HNA is a recommended public health tool to provide evidence about a population on which to plan services and address health inequalities
- HNA provides an opportunity to engage with specific populations and enable them to contribute to targeted service planning and resource allocation
- HNA provides an opportunity for cross-sectoral partnership working and developing creative and effective interventions
- HNA can provide a systematic process for monitoring progress of national and local strategies for actions on health inequalities
- HNA can help to strengthen community involvement in decision-making
- HNA can improve team and partnership working
- HNA can promote professional development
- HNA can improve communication with other agencies and the public
- HNA can improve use of scarce resources

Source: www.publichealth.nice.org

Some authors see needs assessment as only one of several steps in the early stages of programme planning, others argue that needs assessment should be seen as an iterative process, ultimately leading to changes in resource allocation (Ewles and Simnett 2003; Cavanagh and Chadwick 2005). Stevens and Gillam (1998) highlight that patterns of service delivery and programme development in the UK are only weakly related to objectively assessed needs, generally because too much needs assessment is divorced from managers' deadlines and priorities.

What is 'need'?

Bradshaw (1972) identified four main categories of need:

- *Normative need* is need which is identified according to a norm (or set standard); such norms are generally set by experts. Benefit levels, for example, or standards of unfitness in houses, have to be determined according to some criterion.
- *Comparative need* concerns problems which emerge by comparison with others who are not in need. For example, one of the most common uses of this approach has been the comparison of social problems in different areas in order to determine which areas are most deprived.
- *Felt need* is need which people say or feel – that is, need from the perspective of the people who have it.
- *Expressed need* is which can be inferred via people's demand for health services.

One further way to understand the concept of need is to consider the related concepts of supply and demand (see Table 2.2 for definitions). In an ideal world, health systems would be able to cater for every need identified in a population. This need would generate a demand for the appropriate service and the supply of services would meet every demand. There would be no difference between giving people what they need and giving them what they want, and also no under- or over-supply of services. In reality however, demand usually outstrips supply, often leading to the uneven supply of services as health professionals have to prioritize within their given set of resources. It is important therefore that any assessment of need is carried out with knowledge of the local demand and supply of services, so that the provision of uneven services is minimized and issues of equity are considered in all the decisions that are taken about the most appropriate action.

Table 2.2 Need, demand and supply

Need	*Need* in health care is commonly defined as the capacity to benefit. If health needs are to be identified then an effective intervention should be available to meet these needs and improve health. There will be no benefit from an intervention that is not effective or if there are no resources available.
Demand	*Demand* is what patients ask for; it is the needs that most doctors encounter. General practitioners have a key role as gatekeepers in controlling this demand, and waiting lists become a surrogate marker and an influence on this demand.
Supply	*Supply* is the health care provided. This will depend on the interests of health professionals, the priorities of politicians, and the amount of money available.

Source: Wright *et al.* (1998)

Activity 2.1

Why is health needs assessment important for health promotion?

 Feedback

You have learnt that needs assessment is an essential activity in health promotion to ensure that scarce resources are directed at those with most need. It provides a process for assessing the health needs of populations and can be used to facilitate shifts in resources from health care to prevention activities. It is important because health promotion programmes must be based on the best available evidence and on the principles of equity.

What are the features of 'good' needs assessment?

From the outset, needs assessment activities should have clear goals. Among these are: generating awareness; satisfying a mandate; aiding in decision-making or promoting action. In addition the assessment should be explicit about whether it is interested in the whole population, a subset defined by place of residence or community of interest or whether it is attempting to address a public health topic area (e.g. coronary heart disease, immunization). Of course it could be any combination of these things.

Once you have decided this you can then define the aims and objectives for the needs assessment to show what it is you want to find out about whom.

Developing a needs assessment plan is an essential first step to ensure that you make explicit the key questions that you are trying to answer, the sources of information that are required and that plans can be drawn up to secure effective implementation of your findings.

The WHO guide for community nurses (2001) identifies five key steps to be undertaken in needs assessment: profiling; prioritizing; planning; implementing; and evaluating. These steps are used and expanded upon in this chapter to help you think through the logical process of needs assessment activity.

Profiling

This involves the collection of relevant information that can inform you about the state of health and health needs of the population and the analysis of this information to identify major health issues. This will usually involve you in:

- making explicit the characteristics of the population in terms of their age, place of residence and ethnicity;
- describing the health status of the people;
- identifying the local factors that affect their health.

A good needs assessment study will employ a range of sources of data and a range of methods employed to analyse the data. Typically it will include data which can describe the target population and the programmes and services already in place, factors affecting health including behaviour and lifestyle, physical and social environment and genetics. The multi-layered model of factors influencing health has become a familiar and accepted approach to understanding how an individual's health is influenced by social, cultural and environmental conditions and provides a useful framework for thinking about the types of data that will be useful in describing the health of the population and their context.

A needs assessment analysis should answer the question: What are the needs and gaps in services? Programme design should be based on a clear understanding of the size, distribution and nature of the problem or need. How many people have the problem or condition? Where are they located? What are their characteristics?

There are two key ways of gathering this information:

- *Routine sources* which typically include census data; vital statistics (including births and deaths); health and lifestyle data and other data relating to the wider determinants of health. Time-series measures of various outcomes such as poverty, unemployment, crime victimization, drug use, education and employment.
- *Ad hoc studies* where data are not available. In this case you may need to collect new data. The most commonly used data collection method for this purpose is a survey (in which data are collected using questionnaires and/or interviews). Other commonly used methods are focus groups (small group discussions with key stakeholders or informants) and key informant interviews (i.e. interviews with individuals with special inside knowledge about the problem or need and the target population). Whatever data collection method you select (and you will probably use a combination of methods), it is essential that the data be representative or, if not, that you understand the ways in which the data are not representative and attempt to compensate those data with additional data.

While there is often much routine data to draw on to inform all stages of the needs assessment process, good quality local information is often difficult to obtain. Where new information collection is required, attempts should be made to use a combination of approaches. Stevens and Gillam (1998) call for triangulation of data to help tell the story of the population being considered. Information therefore should be considered from routine and ad hoc sources, can be numerical or textual and may sometimes have to be taken from national or regional sources acting as proxy measures for the local situation.

Prioritizing

This involves a process and assessment of four key areas for action:

- What programmes are currently being provided and what is known about the effectiveness of these approaches?
- What do local people see as their health needs?
- What are the national and local priorities for health?
- What is the best available evidence we have to determine the interventions with potential for biggest health gains?

Essentially the prioritizing stage of needs assessment aims to help you reassess current provision of services and programmes against felt need expressed by both professionals and lay people. It also allows you to gather the most up to date knowledge about 'what works' to improve health and reduce health inequalities, and to select those actions most likely to have the biggest impact in terms of health gain.

Planning

This involves selecting and developing the programmes most likely to bring about change and identifying the key stakeholders (who you need to work with and who the programmes that will be developed are targeted at). Including stakeholders in the planning processes will ensure their perspectives are represented, ownership of the needs assessment outcomes is secured and the effectiveness of the actions is guaranteed.

This involves detailing the steps that will be put in place to bring about change and ultimately shifts in resources to those with most need. All action plans should endeavour to be transparent in terms of the process. This will involve being clear about:

• what it is you are trying to achieve and how you are going to do it (aims and objectives);
• where you are now (baseline measures);
• how you will know whether you have achieved your aims and objectives (monitoring and evaluation).

Planning is covered in more detail in Chapter 14.

Implementing the planned activities

Over the last decade our knowledge about what works in health promotion has increased and there are an increasing number of international and national organizations (e.g. Centre for Disease Control, Atlanta (www.cdc.gov); Cochrane Collaboration (www.cochrane.org) and the National Institute of Health and Clinical Excellence (www.nice.org.uk)) whose job it is to synthesize and disseminate knowledge about the most effective interventions in health promotion and public health. This knowledge is an essential starting point for those conducting local needs assessment studies. However, there are many issues to consider in the transfer of interventions that those carrying out needs assessment should consider (see Chapter 16).

Evaluation of health outcomes

It is important that all needs assessment studies should involve an evaluation which will allow you to assess what has changed as a result of your profiling, prioritizing, planning and implementing. In some ways evaluations take you back to the start as they allow you to reassess where you are now and the process starts again. The evaluation usually asks the questions: What worked well? What problems were encountered? How could you have done it better? Once the evaluation is complete, share it with others interested in needs assessments. This will provide an opportunity to learn from one another (see Chapter 15).

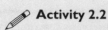

Activity 2.2

What are the key features of the five stages of needs assessment outlined above and what challenges do most professionals face in carrying out each stage?

Feedback

Profiling	• Good use of routine and other sources of information to describe the size and characteristics of the population • Populations should be described in terms of geography, setting, social experience (e.g. age group ethnicity etc.) and experience of a particular medical condition • A broad definition of the determinants of health should be used to describe the population
Prioritizing	• Use of explicit criteria for prioritizing actions, including an assessment of which determinants of the biggest impact on the burden of illness and which interventions have the most potential to see improvements in health • Decisions on priorities should be balanced to match national priorities and the views of local people
Planning	• Aims and objectives of the needs assessment exercise should be clear; roles and responsibilities of those involved in interventions made explicit; resources identified for all aspects of the implementation and evaluation process
Implementation	• Choose realistic timescales for the delivery of the intervention • Be clear about some of the barriers to effective implementation and put in place actions to overcome these barriers • Put in place mechanisms to ensure ongoing and effective consultation with users
Evaluation	• Process and outcome indicators should be used to assess the effectiveness of your programme • A combination of methods should be used to assess the success of your interventions (e.g. quantitative and qualitative data) • Methods chosen should be driven by the purpose of the evaluation

Tackling health inequalities – needs assessment, health equity auditing and other tools and techniques

Many countries of Europe are richer and healthier than they have ever been before. However, health inequalities remain a key challenge for many governments across Europe and internationally. Encouragingly, over the last 10–15 years there has been a substantial increase both in the recognition of the existence of inequalities and the development of a range of policies aimed at reducing them. Documenting inequalities has become common. What is less common at a service level is the clear targeting of resources to identified needs and reviewing the impact of interventions designed to reduce inequalities in health. Having a better picture of the inequalities that exist helps to target resources at those in greatest need.

Programmes designed to reduce inequalities often fail due to the time and resources available to carry them out and a lack of evidence about what works across different segments of the population. Increased policy commitment internationally to tackle health inequalities has led some governments to introduce mandatory systems for assessing need against all aspects of health inequalities.

In England for example, the concept of health equity auditing (HEA) has been introduced to ensure that local community plans for health and development prioritize those with the greatest need. HEA identifies how fairly services or other resources are distributed in relation to the health needs of different groups and areas, and the priority action to provide services relative to need. Unlike some needs assessments, HEA is not complete until something changes to reduce health inequalities, for example, changes in resource allocation, commissioning, service provision or health outcomes.

HEA provides a framework for systematic action. It highlights the need to think about inequalities in terms of age, gender, disability, geography and disability as well as socioeconomic status. An HEA will consider the health needs of particular groups taking account of at least one of these dimensions against the provision of services and resources for good health.

There are six stages in HEA: stage 1 – agree priorities and partners; stage 2 – do an equity profile, identify the gap; stage 3 – agree high impact local action to narrow the gap; stage 4 – agree priorities for action; stage 5 – secure changes in investment and service delivery; stage 6 – review progress and assess impact.

You should note at this stage that the overall process of HEA is not dissimilar to the process of a 'gold standard' needs assessment. Some argue it is just a new fashionable way of describing needs assessment processes with a particular emphasis on the issue of health inequalities. Hamer *et al.* (2003) indeed admit that HEA is not new and that NHS organizations, local authorities and other agencies have been working for many years to identify and reduce inequalities in the health and well-being of different groups in their communities. However, they stress that the difference now is that tackling health inequalities is integrated into mainstream planning and service delivery within the NHS and partner agencies and has become mandatory in England.

Hamer *et al.* argue that there are a number of ways in which a health equity audit can assess equity in service delivery in the NHS, local government or elsewhere. This can include a review of:

- *equal access for equal need*: such as greater availability of free fruit in schools in the most deprived areas;
- *equal use for equal need*: such as greater use of smoking cessation services among low-income smokers;
- *equal quality of care for all*: such as culturally appropriate and relevant maternity services for black and minority ethnic communities;
- *equal outcomes for equal need*: such as greater reductions in coronary heart disease mortality among lower socioeconomic groups.

Health impact assessment (HIA), which you will learn about in Chapter 13, is also used as a tool for decision-makers in assessing health inequalities in local populations. The purpose of HIA is to identify the potential health consequences of a proposal on a given population and to maximize the positive health benefits and minimize potential adverse effects on health and inequalities.

HIA has been in existence much longer than the concept of HEA in its formal sense and is gaining increasing importance on the international stage as a key tool for health promotion decision-making.

Quigley *et al.* (2005) compare the similarities and differences of HEA and HIA along with other techniques such as integrated impact assessment and race equality impact assessment. In doing so, they attempt to highlight their unique contribution to assessing health needs, informing decisions and assessing impact.

The commonality between these approaches is that they are all used as planning tools to promote decision-making to ensure effective public health services, in both the health and non-health sectors and that they all work best when they involve a wide variety of stakeholders, building new ways of working together and ensuring joined-up planning – at project, programme, strategy or policy levels.

Activity 2.3

Describe the main differences between the complementary techniques of health needs assessment, HEA and HIA and find examples to illustrate your answer. In your view, how different are these techniques and do these differences warrant the investment in their development?

Feedback

All three approaches can be used to take account of inequalities to help improve health and reduce health inequalities:

- HNA by providing a local picture of inequalities through describing the health needs and health assets of different groups within the population
- HIA by viewing how proposals may affect the most vulnerable groups in the population compared with how they may affect the least vulnerable
- HEA by redirecting investment in organizational resources to places where there is most inequity

HNA, HIA, and HEA can then tailor recommendations to address inequalities – for example by changing priorities and targeting resources – or at least ensure inequalities do not widen further. Their common features include:

- improve health, especially inequalities, and promote social justice
- have both short and long timescales, and avoid compromising the health of future generations
- require broad ownership and involvement of the target population
- require real collaboration of all key players
- are systematic, explicit and transparent
- use the social model of health, although HNA also includes the medical model
- require a wide range of skills, knowledge and experience
- require a wide range of types and sources of information
- require a balance between the time taken to undertake the assessment and the potential benefits

(www.publichealth.nice.org)

Community involvement, asset mapping and needs assessment

In recent years, there has been greater recognition of the importance of social factors in the aetiology of health and disease with an increase in public health strategies which set out proposals to tackle health inequalities. Although there is a dearth of rigorous evaluations of social interventions aimed at reducing health inequalities, reviews have identified certain characteristics of successful approaches (Gillies 1997; NHS Centre for Reviews and Dissemination 1997):

- local assessment of needs, especially involving local people in the research process itself;
- mechanisms that enable organizations to work together – ensuring dialogue, contact and commitment;
- representation of local people within planning and management arrangements – the greater the level of involvement, the larger the impact;
- design of specific initiatives with target groups to ensure that they are acceptable (i.e. culturally and educationally appropriate), and that they work through settings that are accessible and appropriate;
- training and support for volunteers, peer educators and local networks, thus ensuring maximum benefit from community-based initiatives;
- visibility of political support and commitment;
- reorientation of resource allocation to enable systematic investment in community-based programmes;
- policy development and implementation that brings about wider changes in organizational priorities and policies, driven by community-based approaches;
- increased flexibility of organizations, so supporting increased delegation and a more responsive approach.

Most people working with local populations realize that good community capacity is a necessary condition for the development, implementation and maintenance of effective interventions and this is reflected in an increasing number of public health strategy documents. However, Jordan *et al.* (1998) argue that while the nature and extent of public involvement in determining health needs has increased, the quality of consultation remains questionable. One reason for this is that policy-makers under heavy pressure to achieve very specific national policy targets may feel that the involvement of the community is time-consuming and that they can suffer a loss of control. This can lead to community involvement activities becoming tokenistic and separated from the main decision-making processes of professionals.

Another problem associated with poor community involvement is that professionals tend to define communities by their deficiencies and needs. These needs are often translated into deficiency-orientated policies and programmes which identify the problems and try to address them. Deficit models tend to define communities and individuals in negative terms, identify problems and needs requiring external actors, measure risk exposure and vulnerability and ask communities to prove that they are worse off than others in order to justify the expenditure of resources – decreasing self-esteem. A possible downside to this approach is highlighted by Kretzmann and McKnight (1993), who claim from their work with communities that many low-income urban neighbourhoods have become environments of service where behaviours are affected because residents come to believe that their well-being depends upon being a client. They therefore suggest that rather than focus on deficits an alternative approach would be to develop policies and activities based on the assets, capabilities and skills of people and their neighbourhoods: 'Communities have never been built upon their deficiencies. Building community has always depended upon mobilising the capacities and assets of a people and a place. That is why a map of neighbourhood assets is necessary if local people are to find the way toward empowerment and renewal'. Asset models tend to accentuate positive ability, capability and capacity to identify problems and activate solutions, which promote the self-esteem of individuals and communities leading to less reliance on professional services.

Opportunities for health protection and promotion are, to a large extent, dependent on local circumstances and assets. The WHO European Office for Investment for Health Development has defined 'health assets' as resources that individuals and communities have at their disposal, which protect against negative health outcomes and/or promote health status. These assets can be social, financial, physical or human resources (e.g. education, employment skills, supportive social networks, natural resources etc.) (Morgan *et al.* 2004).

An inventory of health and development assets would, as a minimum, include family and friendship (supportive) networks, intergenerational solidarity, community cohesion, environmental resources necessary for promoting physical, mental and social health, employment security and opportunities for voluntary service, affinity groups (e.g. mutual aid), religious tolerance and harmony, lifelong learning, safe and pleasant housing, political democracy and participation opportunities, social justice and enhancing equity.

Ziglio *et al.* (2000) maintain that thinking in terms of assets for health and development does not come naturally. Most interventions to promote health ought to focus on the needs or problems of a population. In most cases this is necessary but not sufficient for bringing about sustainable and equitable results. An effective and sustainable strategy for health will also require the strengthening of individual and community health and development assets. In other words, need reduction must be complemented by action, tailored to maximize the health and development assets present in a given country or community.

The identification and strengthening of health-promoting assets will help to achieve equity in promoting health, strengthening community involvement, stimulating intersectoral collaboration and defining health's role in economic and social development.

An asset-based approach to health and development adds value to the deficit model by:

- promoting the population as a co-producer of health rather than simply a consumer of health care services, thus reducing the demand on scarce resources;
- strengthening the capacity of individuals and communities to realize their potential for contributing to health development;
- contributing to more equitable and sustainable social and economic development and hence the goals of other sectors.

Good health needs assessment should provide a means of identifying the health assets and needs of a given population to inform decisions about service delivery in order to improve health and reduce health inequalities.

Learning how to ask what communities have to offer begins a process of building and developing. It brings knowledge, skills and capacities out into the open, where they can work together to everyone's benefit. As the web of assets grows, so does the potential for the community.

Kretzmann and McKnight (1993) have described a useful way (through 'asset mapping') of measuring and diagnosing positive community capacity prior to intervening, which helps focus activity on the areas requiring attention and thus ensures more successful project implementation. An asset map is an inventory of the strengths and gifts of the people who make up a community. Asset mapping reveals the assets of the entire community and highlights the interconnections among them, which in turn reveals how to access those assets.

The community asset mapping process is intended to initiate a process that will fully mobilize a community to use its assets around a vision and a plan to solve its own problems. Kretzmann and McKnight illustrate the differences between the traditional approach to assessing need and the assets approach which identifies the following distinct categorizations for asset identification:

- *primary building blocks* – assets and capacities located inside the neighbourhood and largely under neighbourhood control (e.g. skills, talents and experience of residents, citizen associations etc.);
- *secondary building blocks* – assets located within the community but largely controlled by outsiders (physical resources such as vacant land, energy and waste resources, public institutions and services);
- *potential building blocks* – resources originating outside the neighbourhood controlled by outsiders (e.g. public capital improvement expenditures).

The needs assessment map (Figure 2.1) and the assets map (Figure 2.2) illustrate the differences taken by professionals to identify needs and develop actions to support the development of healthy communities. Guy *et al.* (2002) promote asset mapping as a positive, realistic (starting with what the community has) and inclusive approach to building the strengths of local communities towards health improvements for all. Assets maps provide a starting point for taking action in a way which builds trust between professionals and local communities.

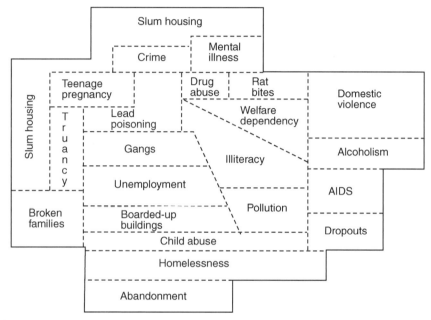

Figure 2.1 Needs assessment map

Source: McKnight (1995)

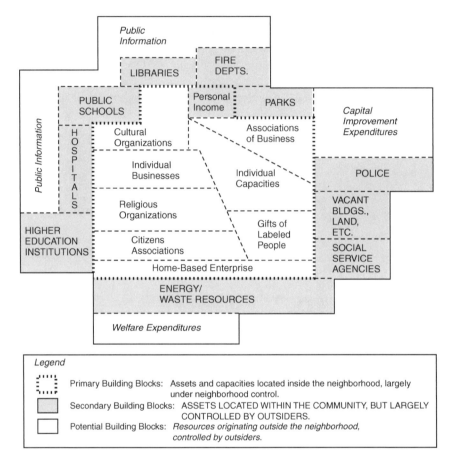

Figure 2.2 Neighbourhood assets map

Source: McKnight (1995)

The concept of asset mapping combined with more traditional ways of measuring need provides health promoters with a potentially more effective way of developing programmes that aim to improve health and tackle health inequalities.

In reality, both models are important. However, more work needs to be done to redress the balance between the more dominant deficit model and the less well known (and understood) assets model. What is needed now is a more robust evidence base which can demonstrate that investing in the assets of individuals, communities and organizations has the potential to develop cost-effective health promotion strategies for the future.

Activity 2.4

Describe the main features of an assets map and contrast the asset mapping approach to that of a traditional needs assessment.

Feedback

Your answer should draw on the work of Kretzman and McKnight to illustrate how the process of asset mapping can help to build strong partnerships between health professionals and the local community – identifying ways in which the community can be involved in all aspects of the planning, development, implementation and evaluation of programmes for health improvement.

Creating a map of the community's assets starts the process of community involvement in health by identifying the gifts, talents and abilities of individuals, associations and institutions. These will be carried out on an ongoing basis and will include information relating to:

- the talents of local residents (including new people who have moved to the community);
- the 'emerging leaders' that can be found in the community
- local institutions, including their physical, human and financial assets
- informal community and neighbourhood organizations
- existing community leaders who are committed to using the gifts and talents of local people, institutions and informal organizations to build a stronger, more vibrant community

Asset mapping is more than an inventory of the skills, talents and resources of individuals and organizations – in order to be effective it should find effective strategies for linking the various talents and resources together.

Summary

Needs assessment in health promotion is essential in the development of appropriate policy and programmatic solutions to public health concerns. It encompasses reviews of health issues, identification and agreement of the priorities for action and demonstration of the most efficient and cost-effective use of scarce resources in the public sector.

Health needs assessment promotes and helps to ensure that those in most need have equal chances of accessing and benefiting from the services and programmes that health promotion provides. It draws on a range of tools and techniques such as health impact assessment, health equity auditing and asset mapping to ensure that programmes are planned, implemented and evaluated in the most efficient way. Needs assessments that are carried out as an integral part of health promotion planning processes can support the most efficient use of scarce resources and support cost-effective approaches to achieving an equitable and sustainable rise in the general level of population health and well-being.

References

Bradshaw J (1972) A taxonomy of social need. *New Society*, March: 640–3.
Cavanagh S, Chadwick K (2005) *Health Needs Assessment: a practical guide.* London: National Institute of Health and Clinical Excellence.

Ewles L, Simnett I (2003) Identifying health promotion needs and priorities. Chapter 6 in *Promoting Health: a practical guide*. London: Baillière Tindall.

Gillies P (1997) Effectiveness of alliances and partnerships for health promotion. *Health Promotion International*, 13: 99–120.

Guy T, Fuller D, Pletsch C (2002) *Asset Mapping: a handbook*. Ottawa, Ontario: Canadian Rural Partnership (available at www.rural.gc.ca/conference/documents/mapping_e.phtml).

Hamer L, Jacobson B, Flowers J, Johnstone F (2003) *Health Equity Audit Made Simple: a briefing for primary care trusts and local strategic partnerships*. Working document. London: Health Development Agency and Public Health Observatories.

Jordan J, Dowswell T, Harrison S, Lilford RJ, Mort M (1998) Health needs assessment: Whose priorities? Listening to the users and the public, *British Medical Journal*, 316: 1668–70.

Kretzmann J, McKnight J (1993) *Building Communities from the Inside Out: a path towards building and mobilising a communities assets*. Evanston, IL: Institute for Policy Research.

McKnight J (1995) *The Careless Society: Community and its counterfeits*. New York: Basic Books.

Morgan A, Ziglio Z, Harrison D, Levin L (2004) *Assets for Health and Development. Overview document: making the case*. European Office for Investment for Health and Development. Venice: WHO.

NHS Centre for Reviews and Dissemination (1997) *Review of Effectiveness of Interventions Aimed at Reducing Inequalities in Health*. York: University of York.

Quigley R, Cavanagh S, Harrison D, Taylor L, Pottle M (2005) *Clarifying Approaches To: health needs assessment, health impact assessment, integrated impact assessment, health equity audit, and race equality impact assessment*. London: Health Development Agency.

Stevens A, Gillam S (1998) Needs assessment from theory to practice, *British Medical Journal*, 316: 1448–52.

WHO (World Health Organization) (2001) *Community Health Needs Assessment: an introductory guide for the family health nurse in Europe*. Copenhagen: WHO.

Wright J, Williams R, Wilkinson J (1998) Development and importance of health needs assessment, *British Medical Journal*, 316: 1310–13.

Ziglio E, Hagard S, McMahon L Harvey S, Levin L (2000) Increasing investment for health: progress so far. Fifth Global conference on health promotion in Mexico, 5–9 June.

Further reading

Peterson D, Alexander G (2001) *Needs Assessment in Public Health – a practical guide for students and professionals*. New York: Kluwer Academic /Plenum Publishers.

3 Reviewing the evidence base for health promotion planning

Overview

The aim of this chapter is to outline some basic approaches to searching and critically appraising research evidence that can provide health promotion planners with some of the information that they require, as well as to discuss the complexities inherent in seeking and appraising different kinds of research evidence. Awareness of this complexity should lead you first to ask whether others have already produced reliable reviews of research that you can use. To help you work through the following learning objectives, the chapter will use scenarios relating to sexual health promotion.

Learning objectives

After reading this chapter, you will be better able to:

- specify a research question
- identify the broad type of research most likely to answer that question
- outline the potential role of systematic reviews of research evidence for health promotion planning and ways of locating and appraising such reviews
- explain the challenges involved in locating and appraising relevant and reliable research evidence for health promotion planning
- describe how existing research evidence is valuable as one part of the jigsaw of information and judgement needed for health promotion planning

Key terms

Acceptability Whether an intervention is acceptable to the recipients or those providing it.

Critical appraisal The consistent assessment of research studies in order to determine the validity or trustworthiness of the evidence they contain.

Effectiveness The extent to which an intervention produces a beneficial result under usual circumstances.

Feasibility A characteristic of issues for which there is a practical solution.

Free-text terms Inconsistently applied terms taken from the text of a reference, used to catalogue research studies.

Indexing (thesaurus) terms Consistently applied database-specific terms used to catalogue research studies.

Outcome evaluation Research that determines the end results of an intervention.

Process evaluation Evaluation that concentrates on examining the process of an intervention.

Search filter A combination of index and free-text terms designed to search a database in order to locate every possible and yet relevant research study.

Systematic review A review of the literature that uses an explicit approach to searching, selecting and combining the relevant studies.

Views study Research that asks and reports on people's perspectives, opinions, beliefs or attitudes about a topic of interest (such as a particular intervention or social exclusion).

Introduction

Using empirical research to inform health promotion planning is a complex experience. There is no simple divide provided by research between 'effective' and 'ineffective' interventions, for a variety of reasons. The relevant evaluation research might just not exist and what research there is may be of varying quality. There may also be differences between the situation you are planning for and the populations, settings or outcomes addressed in the existing research studies. As well as asking whether an intervention has been shown to be effective or not, we must also look at its likely feasibility and acceptability. Judgements need to be made about the likelihood that interventions found to be feasible, acceptable and/or effective in one setting will be so in another.

Moving from a planning need to a researchable question

Working through the activities in Chapter 2, you will have thought about the particular health need present in your setting and the health promotion planning that is required to meet that need. What is now required is for you to reframe your health need into researchable questions. As later sections will show, this will help you avoid being overwhelmed by the quantity and range of research that you are likely to come into contact with.

Research evidence can be used to identify likely causal or modifying factors for health and disease, and identify the likely range or extent of needs in given populations. However, this chapter concentrates instead on using existing research to evaluate the potential for particular health promotion interventions to address such needs.

Evaluation research questions and helpful study designs

Various types of questions can be asked about health promotion interventions, including those relating to *effectiveness, feasibility* and *acceptability*. While these concepts may tend to overlap to some extent, here each one is looked at in turn.

An intervention's *effectiveness* is sometimes defined as whether it works to help produce favourable outcomes. Others talk in terms of an overall balance of benefit and harm. After all, there are numerous aspects of life that might be influenced and, even with the best intentions, it is possible to have a negative influence as well as a positive one. For example, a health education intervention aiming to reduce unintended pregnancies among adolescents might also bring benefits in terms of reduced rates of sexually transmitted infections and self-esteem. However, such an intervention could also potentially bring about harms, for example to the self-esteem of those adolescents who are already pregnant or parents.

If looking for answers about effectiveness, you will therefore need to identify studies that evaluate outcomes, both positive and negative, after exposure to an intervention. The various designs that attempt this can be grouped together under the umbrella term 'outcome evaluation'. It is widely but not universally held that experimental designs, in particular randomized controlled trials (RCTs), are superior to other kinds of design for determining a causal relation between an intervention and its intended outcomes. These designs allocate study participants so that some receive an intervention and some do not. If allocation is done at random, it is argued, the baseline characteristics of study participants should not have led to any differences in outcomes between the two groups and any difference seen can be attributed instead to the intervention. However, due to issues of practicality and ethics, experimental studies are not always possible. For this and other reasons they can be in short supply and other designs may need to be considered. These include designs that compare recipients of an intervention with others drawn from the general population or from groups matched on certain baseline characteristics (sometimes called controlled before and after designs), or studies that repeatedly examine outcomes within one group over time (e.g. interrupted time-series designs).

It may be that you are satisfied that a health promotion intervention is effective but instead want to consider whether it will be *feasible* in your own setting. You will want to explore what is known about the circumstances or processes that help an intervention to work or impede effectiveness. In reading existing studies of interventions you might want to know, for example:

- How was the intervention developed or modified (e.g. what was the nature of participatory work with potential intervention recipients and providers)?
- What was the intervention's planned content (e.g. activities, materials, media and settings) and the intensity of contact between the intervention and those receiving it?
- What actually happened (e.g. who did the intervention reach, which providers were actually involved in delivery, which intervention components were actually delivered, what did those involved in providing the intervention have to say about how it was implemented and what were the financial, time and other resource costs)?

While this kind of evidence about intervention processes can be produced as an integral part of studies that also evaluate outcomes, such process evaluations can also be stand-alone. In either case, a variety of data collection methods can be employed such as questionnaires, observations, interviews and focus groups, with or without comparison between groups of people or over time.

When seeking evidence about an intervention's *acceptability*, emphasis is often placed upon the views or experiences of the public or service users; that is, people likely to be at the receiving end of interventions. Again there is no single study design through which evidence about acceptability should be produced. Participants in experimental studies of intervention outcomes can also be asked for feedback about their experiences, as can people questioned in non-experimental intervention studies. In building up a picture of how one might appropriately intervene in people's lives, it might even be helpful to find evidence of people's views about important influences in their lives. These may be located in local or population-based questionnaires, interviews or focus-group studies that are conducted independently of any intervention evaluation.

Specifying the other dimensions of your research question

Having clarified whether you are interested in effectiveness, feasibility, acceptability or all three, and having thought about study designs that might help you answer your question type, you then need to specify the other dimensions of your research question. In doing this it will help to define the boundaries of your interest as explicitly as you can.

For example, if you are interested in an intervention's effectiveness you would normally build your question by focusing in turn on three dimensions of study: the population; the intervention; and the outcomes of interest. One example of an effectiveness question is: 'In females aged 11–16 years, do educational or career development interventions have an effect on the rate of unintended teenage pregnancy?' This question indicates clearly that interest is focused on younger teenage or even pre-teen women, on two types of social intervention and on a particular type of pregnancy. You can probably already see how some of these terms need to be specified further. Before progressing much further, for example, you should probably specify what kinds of pregnancy you would consider as 'unintended'.

Again, using the idea of a question structured according to population, intervention and outcomes, a question about feasibility of implementation might be phrased thus: 'What are the ethnicities and ages of the young people actually reached by voluntary service programmes for vulnerable teenagers aimed at preventing teenage pregnancy?' An acceptability question might focus either on a specific intervention or on a health area, while also specifying a population and the kinds of views of interest. Examples include: 'What kinds of interventions do young parents regard as important and appropriate influences on their lives as teenage parents?' and 'What are the perspectives of young people in the UK on the role of social exclusion in teenage pregnancy?'

Activity 3.1

> Select a health promotion intervention you are interested in and draft one research question each about the intervention's effectiveness, feasibility and acceptability. Then think about the kinds of research designs that might help you address each of these questions, taking five minutes to complete each question.

 Feedback

> You may have chosen to specify your questions very precisely or instead opted for a broader focus in some or all of the defining dimensions, perhaps along the lines of: 'I'd like to know the extent to which various health promotion interventions are effective (and/or feasible and/or acceptable) for affecting this problem'. The broader your research question's focus, the more likely it is that research exists to answer it. However, as much of this chapter will illustrate, a broad focus also means more work. The broader the question, for example, the more potentially relevant research you will have to screen to find the research you actually want.

This section has explained the importance of thinking through the kind of research you are really interested in before you start to look. Identifying these different research dimensions should also help you when the searching and appraising actually starts.

Locating relevant research

The breadth of research literature available to inform policy and planning is staggering. Busy policy-makers and practitioners in public health will rarely have the time to find and assess all of this research evidence.

Probably the best step to take before starting searches in any depth is to seek out an information specialist or librarian and ask their advice. Librarians should be able to guide you as to which bibliographic databases might be best suited for your needs, and can help with drawing up sets of search terms and with the tricky act of running searches on databases. They can also help you identify other potential sources to search (e.g. health promotion journals held by local libraries that might not be indexed well or at all by databases).

The next essential step is to ensure you don't reinvent the wheel. You should look to see whether anyone has already summarized and appraised research for the topic you are interested in. Several international initiatives are now underway that focus upon the production and dissemination of high quality reviews of research of relevance to health promotion, as will be seen below.

Examples of sources that provide access to reviews of health promotion research evidence and to health research are listed in Table 3.1.

Table 3.1 Sources of health promotion and public health research

	Scope	Access details	How to search	Advantages/disadvantages
Sources of systematic reviews				
Effective Public Health Practice Project (EPHPP)	Conducts systematic reviews on the effectiveness of public health interventions, and summarizes recent, high quality reviews produced by others	www.city.hamilton.on.ca/PHCS/EPHPP/	By scanning the titles of completed reviews and summaries of reviews	Evidence in the reviews is already critically appraised and synthesized
The Community Guide (Guide to Community Preventive Services)	Reviews and assesses the quality of available evidence on the 'effectiveness and cost-effectiveness of essential community preventive health services'. Broad public health focus	www.thecommunityguide.org/	By scanning the titles of completed reviews	Some provide access to the full review (Cochrane Library, DARE)
The EPPI-Centre Database of Promoting Health Effects Reviews (DoPHER)	A specialized register concentrating on reviews of effectiveness in health promotion and public health, identified as a result of conducting systematic reviews within the EPPI-Centre. It was last updated to December 2003 and work is currently in progress to update it to January 2005	http://eppi.ioe.ac.uk/EPPIWeb/home.aspx?&page=/hp/databases.htm	Using a free-text or controlled vocabulary. Each review is coded according to type of research, country, health focus, population, and quality assessment criteria	For some databases, access to bibliographic details is free for those with web access (Cochrane Library, DARE, DoPHER)
				Reviews may meet a minimum standard of quality (Cochrane Library and DARE) or those of a higher quality may be identifiable (DoPHER)
Public Health Electronic Library (PheL)	Aims to provide knowledge and knowhow to promote health, prevent disease and reduce health inequalities. Posts evidence documents produced by the Centre for Public Health Evidence at the National Institute for Health and Clinical Excellence (NICE), including evidence briefings and evidence reviews	www.phel.gov.uk/	By scanning the titles of completed reviews and summaries	Controlled vocabulary of Cochrane Library and DARE rely on MeSH terms, which may

Source	Description	Website/access	Searching	Limitations
The Cochrane Database of Systematic Reviews (CDSR)	Regularly updated collection of systematic reviews in evidence-based medicine	www.cochrane.org/reviews/index.htm abstracts free; full text by subscription (arranged nationally in some countries, e.g. via National Electronic Library for Health in UK)	Using MeSH terms from MEDLINE or free-text. Examples include 'health promotion', 'health education', 'primary prevention', 'preventative health services'	make it more difficult to find reviews relevant to health promotion and public health
Database of Reviews of Effectiveness (DARE)	Summaries of systematic reviews which have met strict quality criteria. Included reviews have to be about the effects of interventions. Each summary also provides a critical commentary on the quality of the review. Covers a broad range of health and social care topics	www.york.ac.uk/inst/crd/crddatabases.htm	Using MeSH terms from MEDLINE as above	The EPPI-Centre's DoPHER is specific to health promotion and public health and uses health promotion specific controlled vocabulary for easy retrieval
Health Technology Assessment (HTA) monographs	Contains research on health care technology assessments. As well as systematic reviews, the database contains ongoing and completed research based on trials, questionnaires and economic evaluations	www.york.ac.uk/inst/crd/htahp.htm	By scanning the titles of completed reviews and summaries	Some sites are not health promotion specific (Cochrane Library, DARE, HTA)

Selected sources of outcome evaluations, process evaluations and views research

Source	Description	Website/access	Searching	Limitations
EPPI Centre's BiblioMap database	A database of health promotion research, compiled over a number of years as a result of searching and coding research for inclusion in systematic reviews. It contains approximately 14,000 records at present and is being added to each time a systematic review is completed as well as being updated on a quarterly basis	http://eppi.ioe.ac.uk	Using a free-text or controlled vocabulary. Each review is coded according to type of research, country, health focus, population, and, for studies describing interventions, intervention site, provider and type	Sources catalogue a huge amount of research

Exhaustive searches require considerable skill and knowledge

Do not generally provide free access to full papers |

Table 3.1 *Continued*

	Scope	Access details	How to search	Advantages/ disadvantages
Combined Health Information Database (CHID)	Covers health information and health education resources on ten topics: AIDS, STD, and TB education; complementary and alternative medicine; deafness and communication disorders; diabetes; digestive diseases; kidney and urologic diseases; maternal and child health; medical genetics and rare disorders; and weight control	www.chid.nih.gov	Using controlled vocabulary and free-text terms	Research found is not critically appraised. Limited to published research only Bias towards research published in English, although EMBASE and LILACS have better coverage of non-English journals than MEDLINE
CINAHL	Covers the nursing and allied health literature from 1982 to the present	subscription required www.cinahl.com/	Using controlled vocabulary and free-text terms	
Sociological Abstracts	Abstracts and indexed international sociology literature in sociology and related disciplines in the social and behavioural sciences	subscription required www.csa.com/	Using controlled vocabulary and free-text terms	
The Cochrane Library Controlled Clinical Trials Register (CCTR)	Contains bibliographic information on controlled trials in medicine and allied health	www.cochrane.org	Using free-text or MeSH terms	
Latin American Caribbean Health Sciences Literature (LILACS)	Covers literature related to the health sciences and medicine	http://bases.bireme.br/cgi-bin/ wxislind.exe/iah/online/ ?IsisScript=iah/iah.xis&base= LILACS&lang=i	Using controlled vocabulary or free-text terms	

Database	Description	Access	Search terms
Web of Science	Contains Social Citation Index (SCI), Social Science Citation Index (SSCI), related conference proceedings	http://wos.mimas.ac.uk/ subscription required	Using free-text terms only
PsycInfo	Contains references to wide range of psychological literature	subscription required www.apa.org/psycinfo/	Using a controlled vocabulary. Relevant terms for public health include 'health education', 'primary mental health promotion', 'preventive medicine', 'health behaviour'
MEDLINE/PubMed	MEDLINE is the US National Library of Medicine's 'premier bibliographic database covering the fields of medicine, nursing, dentistry, veterinary medicine, the health care system, and the preclinical sciences'	//www.ncbi.nlm.nih.gov/entrez/query.fcgi?DB=pubmed	Using MeSH terms or free-text terms. Searches can be limited to randomized controlled trials and systematic reviews only
EMBASE	EMBASE, the Excerpta Medica database, is a biomedical and pharmacological database of references from international journals	www.embase.com	Using a set controlled vocabulary known as 'medical descriptors' or free-text terms. Relevant terms for health promotion include 'health promotion', 'health education', 'primary prevention', 'education programme'

Source: adapted from Harden in Oliver and Peersman (2001) and Jackson and Waters (2005)

When planning searches for reviews the following points may be helpful:

- No single source provides access to all the health promotion and public health reviews that exist. This means that you may also want to search other, more general sources too.
- The sources listed vary in terms of how they can be searched. Some, like the Community Guide, are websites that have basic search engines built into them for searching using simple free-text terms, while others are bibliographic databases that use powerful search engines that can run quite complex searches.
- Some databases, for example the Cochrane Database of Systematic Reviews and the Database of Abstracts of Reviews of Effectiveness (DARE), only contain systematic reviews.
- Others, such as the Social Science Research Unit's Database of Promoting Health Effectiveness Reviews (DoPHER) have indexing terms (see below) that can either be applied to identify systematic reviews from a larger pool of reviews, or can be used to identify specific methods that authors may have used to make their reviews more systematic (such as describing their search strategy used to locate primary studies for their review).
- If the source does not catalogue references with the kind of study type used, try limiting your search with terms such as 'systematic review', 'synthesis' or 'meta-analysis' (see below for more detail about review search terms and the possible pitfalls of restricting searches with study-type terms).
- Systematic reviews that address questions of intervention effectiveness far outnumber those addressing other kinds of research question. It is possible, however, for systematic reviews of health promotion to integrate different types of evidence. Some review organizations (e.g. the Cochrane Collaboration) focus solely on questions of effectiveness; others (e.g. the Social Science Research Unit's EPPI-Centre) have a broader focus such as synthesizing research on effectiveness, feasibility and acceptability. Reflecting this, the study types reviewed by different review organizations vary. While Cochrane reviewers, for example, tend to focus on RCTs, EPPI-Centre health promotion reviews draw on controlled trials (with and without random allocation), process evaluations and views studies.
- You will find some reviews that are very highly specified, while others explore broader questions. While a narrow focus can provide clear answers and simplify the research process, its utility may be limited for health promotion policy-makers and service users.
- If you can't find a relevant review that has been published, it is possible that there is one in production or that there are other people out there wanting to start a review. The Cochrane Collaboration's Health Promotion and Public Health Field maintains a list of ongoing health promotion reviews and members interested in different topics. If you have the time and interest to summarize the evidence on your health need, you might want to consider joining a review team and contributing your experience. The Field also provides training and guidance to new and experienced reviewers. For more information on how to become involved, visit www.vichealth.vic.gov.au/cochrane.

Increasingly, reviews of research evidence are being done in ways that attempt to deal with the challenges of making reliable research evidence available to policy-makers, practitioners and the public. Being able to seek out and identify such reviews is an important skill for health promotion planners.

It is worth remembering that research reviews are just as subject to bias in their methods as primary studies. Biases in a review of studies of intervention effectiveness, for example, could lead to conclusions that make an intervention appear more or less effective than it actually is. It is worth considering what might make a review biased and how this might be overcome. These influences are important if we want to appraise the quality of any reviews that we might use to modify policy or practice. They are also clearly important to consider if we are reviewing research ourselves.

Reviews may be adversely affected because they do not contain all of the relevant studies possible. For example, in compiling a review of effectiveness, the easiest studies to find can often be a biased subset. Studies that are published in the most accessible locations, such as in large biomedical databases, like PubMed, can come from journals that tend to avoid publishing inconclusive study results in favour of positive results (International Committee of Medical Journal Editors 2004). Studies reporting non-significant or even negative results are not as likely to be published and are thus more difficult to locate (Easterbrook *et al.* 1991; Hopewell *et al.* 2002). We can also be unintentionally influenced by our own expertise and preferences. Studies which report results that resonate with our own previous experience or beliefs are more likely to be kept on hand.

Using a partial set of studies to answer our research question in these ways may only provide one side, or a distorted image of the evidence picture. Therefore it is important to identify reviews that have searched exhaustively for all relevant literature and have consistently assessed it used pre-specified criteria: these are often the two characteristics used to label a review as being systematic. Health promotion review indexing done by the authors and their colleagues at the EPPI-Centre in the UK specifies that, for a review to be systematic, authors should as a minimum describe which sources they searched for primary studies and what criteria were used to include and exclude primary studies from the review. Once a review has been judged to be systematic, its precise methods should then be critically appraised. Oliver and Peersman (2001) have argued for the use of the criteria shown in Table 3.2 to appraise systematic reviews critically.

Are the results of the review valid?
1 Did the review address a clearly focused issue?
2 Did the authors select the right sort of studies for the review?
3 Do you think the important, relevant studies were included?
4 Did the review's authors do enough to assess the quality of the included studies?
5 Were the results similar from study to study?

What are the results?
6 What is the overall result of the review?
7 How precise are the results?

Will the results help locally?
8 Can the results be applied to the local population?
9 Were all important outcomes considered?
10 Are the benefits worth the harms and costs?

Table 3.2 Quality assessment criteria for reviews

Source: Oliver and Peersman (2001)

Several sources for systematic reviews are listed. Some of them use indexing or thesaurus terms to catalogue the reviews in online databases so they can be searched using either index terms or free-text terms (i.e. BiblioMap, CDSR, DARE), while the remainder of sources list the titles of reviews only, to be scanned manually (e.g. Public Health Effectiveness Project, The Community Guide to Preventive Services, Public Health Electronic Library, Health Technology Assessment Monographs). Similarly, sources of outcome evaluations, process evaluations and views research such as BiblioMap have the ability to be searched online, again using either index terms or free-text terms. Web of Science is the only one of these database sources that allows searching by free-text terms only.

Previous work (Harden *et al.* 1999; Kavanagh *et al.* 2002) offers a number of pointers when planning searches:

- You should complement searches of general databases with searches of health promotion-specific databases.
- Many databases have their own sets of indexing terminology or controlled vocabulary for searching, also known as a 'thesaurus', that you need to get to know if you are going to increase your yield of relevant studies. You can instruct most databases to restrict searches to look solely for references that have been given a particular index term. Again, however, this approach can be problematic, because indexing is inevitably subject to human error. Searches using index terms are often therefore supplemented by free-text searches for the words or phrases that authors might use within the title or abstract.
- There is no such thing as an agreed taxonomy of research designs. As a result, both database indexing and the terms that authors use in their titles and abstracts are not very good at distinguishing between different kinds of research or between research and other kinds of papers. Haphazardly chosen study design or research methods terms can miss potentially relevant research.

These pointers illustrate the complexity involved in just trying to locate the research you are interested in. Before using the above suggestions to embark on a search, it is important to talk through your plans with an information specialist.

A searching technique in particular that it is worth thinking through prior to any such discussion with an information specialist is one where you go back to the structure of your research question and try to think of potential synonyms for each of your question's dimensions. An information specialist can then help you map these terms onto the indexing terms used by the databases you are going to search and use the search engine of the database you are interrogating to combine all of these sets of search terms. If you know of a study that fits your research question it is possible to start this process yourself. You need to take each database in turn and look to see if the study is on it. If it is, you then need to identify which indexing terms the database has applied and consider adding them to your search strategy.

For an effectiveness question, for example you might develop draft sets of terms that are synonyms for your research dimensions of population, intervention and outcome. If you combine sets of search terms in this way, the resulting references will be restricted to those that contain at least one of the selected terms from each set. Figure 3.1 illustrates this approach to searching for a question that is about the effects of health promotion interventions on reducing teenage pregnancy or social exclusion.

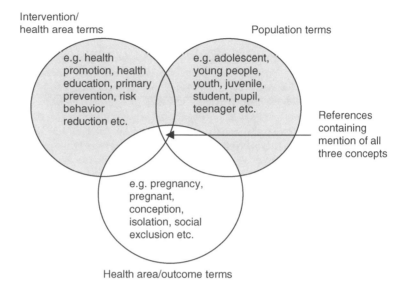

Figure 3.1 Using research questions to focus literature searching

Sets of search terms that together describe a dimension of research are sometimes called 'filters'. These 'search filters' are time-consuming to build and test. However, several groups have developed and tested their own and some of these are freely available. The Centre for Reviews and Dissemination (www.york.ac.uk/inst/crd/search.htm) can provide search filters for systematic reviews in general. The EPPI-Centre can provide a search filter for broad health promotion and public health topics, a filter to locate reviews of effectiveness, as well as several specific topic filters based on past health promotion reviews. Researchers from the National Institute for Health and Clinical Excellence have developed health promotion-specific review search filters for a variety of social science sources (see www.publichealth.nice.org.uk/page.aspx?o=516406).

 Activity 3.2

Using a diagram similar to Figure 3.1, go back to one of the research questions drafted in Activity 3.1 and take 15 minutes to try to brainstorm the various terms that might be used to describe each of the concepts contained within the study. Try to think about ways in which authors might use words or phrases in the abstracts or titles of papers. Try also to apply what knowledge you have about variations in health promotion terminology used in different countries in coming up with relevant terms.

 Feedback

Your diagram will have involved several dimensions, the number depending on whether you selected an effectiveness question or one focused upon feasibility or acceptability. You may have distinguished between terms or even spellings likely to be used by American, Canadian, English or Australian authors, or even have suggested non-English language terms, which would be important if you were keen to explore a method that had been developed and possibly researched in a country that did not use English as its first language. In practice, this kind of brainstorming may only get you so far and an approach that builds on identified search terms might be helpful. You may find, for example, that a paper published in a country that you are not so familiar with, or browsing through available database indexing systems, leads you to other synonyms for the same concept. If you were not able to get very far with this activity you could reflect on whether the dimensions in your research question are sufficiently specified or whether they are still too vague to use in a search. This might also be a good moment to think about what kind of support you might need for this kind of work. Can you identify colleagues that you could do this kind of brainstorming with? How would you go about getting support from information specialists to turn this conceptual work into a practical strategy for searching several databases?

Critically appraising research

Regardless of which type of potentially useful evidence is to be used, once located it must be critically appraised in order to determine if it is valid and useful for your needs. Many guides have been developed to help evaluate the validity or trustworthiness of evidence and different groups advocate different criteria as a way of judging quality. In the absence of consensus, having criteria by which to assess studies can at least provide an explicit and consistent way of looking for indicators of quality across research studies.

Various groups have developed sets of criteria for judging the quality of outcome evaluations (Deeks *et al.* 2003). Oliver and Peersman (2001) describe certain characteristics of studies identified as important for maximizing the validity of findings on intervention effectiveness (Table 3.3).

Are the results of the outcome evaluation valid?
1   Did the evaluation address a clearly focused issue?
2   Were the people receiving the intervention compared with an equivalent control or comparison group?
3   Were all the people who entered the evaluation properly accounted for and attributed at its conclusion?
4   Was the intervention described clearly?
5   Is it clear how the control group and experimental groups did or did not change after the intervention?

What are the results?
6   How large was the impact of the intervention?
7   How precise are the results?

Will the results help me?
8   Can the results be applied to the local population?
9   Were all important outcomes considered?
10 Are the benefits worth the harms and costs?

Table 3.3 Quality assessment criteria for outcome evaluations
Source: Oliver and Peersman (2001)

Criteria for examining the quality of process evaluations have also been developed, but at present little methodological work has been undertaken to determine which criteria are 'best' to use. As a suggested framework (Oliver and Peersman 2001), process evaluation studies assessing implementation have been considered to be of good quality if they meet many or all of the criteria listed in Table 3.4.

Are the results of the process evaluation reliable? Does the study:
1 Focus on a health promotion intervention?
2 Have clearly stated aims?
3 Describe the key processes involved in delivering this intervention?
4 Tell you enough about planning and consultation?
5 Tell you enough about the collaborative effort required for the intervention?
6 Tell you enough about the materials used in the intervention?
7 Tell you enough about how the target population was identified and recruited?
8 Tell you enough about education and training?

What are the results?
9 Were all the processes described and adequately monitored?
10 Was the intervention acceptable?

Will the results help me?
11 Can the results be applied to the local population?
12 Were all important processes considered?
13 If you wanted to know whether this intervention promotes health what outcomes would you want to measure?

Table 3.4 Quality assessment criteria for process evaluations

Source: Oliver and Peersman (2001)

Criteria for judging the quality of studies of people's 'views' have only been developed more recently and one set of criteria is presented in Table 3.5. Harden *et al.* (2001) argue that, in the absence of consensus on what designs and methods should be used in such studies to make them trustworthy, at the very least it is important to understand which designs and research methods such studies used.

---

1 An explicit account of theoretical framework and/or inclusion of a literature review.
2 Clearly stated aims and objectives.
3 Clear description of context.
4 Clear description of sample and sampling methods.
5 Clear description of methodology, including data collection and data analysis methods.
6 Evidence of attempts to establish reliability and validity of data analysis.
7 Inclusion of sufficient original data to mediate between data and interpretation.

Table 3.5 Quality assessment criteria for 'views' studies

Source: Harden *et al.* (2001)

In brief, guidelines exist that will assist in deciding if any primary effectiveness, feasibility or acceptability research located to answer your question was well conducted, or at the least, reported in enough detail to understand whether there was any potential for bias.

Once studies have been located and have been critically appraised against criteria relevant to their research design, what is to be done with them? Should only high quality studies be used or can poorer quality studies be used but somehow given less weight? How do we decide which studies are 'good enough' to be used? At present, studies determined to be of lower quality (i.e. failing more of the questions asked at the critical appraisal stage) tend not to be used to generate conclusions about effectiveness, implementation, feasibility or acceptability. However, they may be used to make recommendations for future research – for testing a promising intervention that was not previously well evaluated, for example.

 Activity 3.3

Read the following two extracts from summaries of systematic reviews. Compare the scope of the two reviews in terms of what kinds of study participants or health promotion methods did studies have to focus on in order to be included.

 HIV prevention programs with heterosexuals (Rotheram-Borus et al. 2000)

Authors' objectives

To identify efficacious human immunodeficiency virus (HIV) prevention programmes designed for heterosexual adults.

Specific interventions included in the review

Studies that aimed to reduce the risk for heterosexual transmission were included. Three types of intervention were identified: those which were based on social cognitive theories that aimed to improve HIV-related knowledge, attitudes, norms and behavioural practices; the treatment of sexually transmitted diseases (STDs); and pre- and post-test HIV testing and counselling programmes.

Participants included in the review

Studies included in the review had to include both men and women or be designed for heterosexual men.

Outcomes assessed in the review

The outcomes included decreases in sexual transmission of HIV following the intervention, the reduction in HIV risk, and the reduction in the rates of STDs.

Study designs of evaluations included in the review

Pre- and post-intervention studies with a comparison condition for heterosexual men and women, or with heterosexual men only, were included.

What sources were searched to identify primary studies?

Index Medicus, Psychological Abstracts, PubMed, MEDLINE and HealthSTAR were searched. In addition, ongoing reviews by government agencies were sought, and interviews were conducted with journal editors and leaders in the field of HIV prevention.

Criteria on which the validity (or quality) of studies was assessed

The authors do not report a method for assessing validity.

How were decisions on the relevance of primary studies made?

The authors do not state how the papers were selected for the review, or how many of the reviewers performed the selection.

How were judgements of validity (or quality) made?

The authors do not state how the papers were assessed for validity, or how many of the reviewers performed the validity assessment.

How were the data extracted from primary studies?

The authors do not state how the data were extracted for the review, or how many of the reviewers performed the data extraction.

Number of studies included in the review

Thirty-two studies with 53,951 participants were included.

How were the studies combined?

The studies were combined narratively within the three main intervention categories described.

How were differences between studies investigated?

The authors did not test for heterogeneity.

 HIV sexual risk reduction interventions for women: a review (Wingood *et al.* 1996)

Authors' objectives

To assess the effectiveness of interventions targeted specifically towards women in increasing condom use during sexual intercourse.

Specific interventions included in the review

Non-theory-based interventions: these typically included single sessions communicating HIV preventive strategies through individual or group counselling or video presentations.

Theoretically-based interventions: these were based on psychological theories, and were typically multi-session programmes that included skills training and strategies to modify perceived peer or partner beliefs about risk-taking behaviour.

Participants included in the review

Women aged from 12 to 40 years, sampled in a range of settings in the US. These included adolescent health, obstetric and primary care clinics, a methadone maintenance programme, a family health centre and an African-American community-based organisation. Studies were excluded if they sampled primarily commercial sex workers. The majority of women in the included in the review were ethnic minority women.

Outcomes assessed in the review

Primarily, reduction in sexual risk behaviours, knowledge, and condom use, though other outcomes are also reported in the appendices.

Study designs of evaluations included in the review

Five randomised controlled trials (RCTs), one non-randomised controlled trial and one before-and-after study were included.

What sources were searched to identify primary studies?

ERIC was searched from 1981 to May 1995, PsycLIT from 1984 to May 1995, and MEDLINE from 1981 to May 1995. The search strategies are provided.

Criteria on which the validity (or quality) of studies was assessed

A set of methodological criteria was used to assess the primary studies. The criteria were: (1) clear description of study site and sample; (2) clear specification of aims; (3) specification of a theoretical framework; (4) description of programme implementation; (5) description of content and behaviour change techniques, sufficiently detailed to permit replication; (6) clear description of differences in treatment and control conditions for primary and secondary outcomes post-intervention; (7) inclusion of a randomly-assigned control or comparison condition; (8) specification of the length of follow-up; (9) specification of refusal rates reported for each study condition; (10) use of blinding; (11) reporting of retention rates for each study condition; (12) adherence to intention-to-treat principles in the data analysis; (13) assessment of pre-test equivalence on sociodemographic, behavioural and psychosocial factors between study conditions; (14) clear description of data analysis techniques; (15) specification of a measure of variability for the designated effect size; and (16) sample size justification.

How were decisions on the relevance of primary studies made?

The papers were assessed for relevance by two independent authors.

How were judgements of validity (or quality) made?

The papers were assessed for validity by two independent authors, and any disagreements were resolved by discussion.

How were the data extracted from primary studies?

The authors do not state how the data were extracted for the review, or how many of the authors performed the data extraction.

Number of studies included in the review

Five RCTs (697 participants), 1 non-randomised trial (214 participants), and 1 before-and-after trial (241 participants) were included.

How were the studies combined?

The studies were combined by a narrative review.

How were differences between studies investigated?

Differences between the studies are described in terms of methodology and whether or not the interventions were theory-based. In addition, the characteristics of the studies in which the intervention proved effective are compared with the characteristics of those in which the intervention was ineffective.

Feedback

You might have noticed that:

- One of the reviews was restricted to studies conducted in the USA alone. Much evaluation research is conducted in the USA and concerns are frequently raised as to possible differences between the social norms seen in the USA and elsewhere. Reviews that include studies from a variety of locations could provide an opportunity to explore these concerns empirically.
- The review foci are quite different in terms of the kinds of participants covered. One review restricted its focus in terms of gender (studies of women only) but also in terms of how participants were recruited (largely through health care settings) and excluded studies of commercial sex workers and interventions targeted at reducing injecting drug behaviours increasing risk of HIV infection. Reviewers explained in their report that this was in order to ensure that the recommendations were applicable to the majority of women at risk of HIV infection. The other review makes no restriction by gender but instead makes restrictions in terms of who was involved in the interventions studied.
- One review required that studies measure distal outcomes relating to disease states or behaviour ('risky sexual behaviour', the transmission of HIV and other sexually transmitted diseases) while the other also included studies of impacts on intermediate measures, such as sexual health knowledge. Other potentially important outcomes, such as impacts on self-reports of perceived control over sexual health, or skills to increase negotiation or in other ways reduce sexual exposure to disease, could have been measured but were not.

If you are interested in examining the strength of research evidence for health promotion, then the relatively methodological abstracts produced by DARE should be of interest to you. Research evidence is also increasingly available in formats designed to be more accessible to practitioners and planners (see e.g. CRD's free publication, *Effectiveness Matters*, available via their website at www.york.ac.uk/inst/crd/em.htm or on written request).

Evidence as one piece of health promotion planning

Existing evidence may be able to provide you with information about how feasible, acceptable and/or effective an intervention *was* in the setting in which its evaluation occurred. You will need to decide what this evidence can tell you about whether such an intervention *will be* feasible, acceptable and/or effective in your own setting. It can't be assumed that these aspects of an intervention are automatically generalizable or transferable from one setting and time to others. You will need to use judgement, informed but not dictated by evidence, to decide to what extent they can be transferred.

Health promotion researchers are just beginning to think about such questions, which they term 'technology transfer'. This stresses the importance of whether an intervention will be feasible, achieve high coverage and be acceptable in another setting and whether an intervention's aims address the needs that are key to promoting health in another setting. When reviewing existing evidence in order to inform action in a new setting, it is important to stress that there is no straight-forward means of synthesizing evidence to produce a simple answer about whether an intervention should be implemented in a new setting. Human judgement is necessary.

 Activity 3.4

Read the two structured abstracts again and reflect on the extent to which you think the health promotion interventions focused upon in these reviews might fit in the health promotion settings you are most familiar with.

 Feedback

You might want to consider aspects of your own setting that would influence these interventions:

- What are the characteristics and needs of your local population?
- Would the interventions be provided by the professionals or volunteers, and would the recipients of the interventions have a preference?
- What kind of funding is available? Would it be enough to finance these interventions?
- Would your organization's management support interventions such as these?

Understanding more about the context within which you want to implement an intervention will help you to decide if it is likely to work.

Summary

Research evidence is increasingly being used to inform health promotion planning. Answering questions about whether an intervention is effective, feasible or acceptable is a complex process. A vast array of literature exists which can be difficult for busy health promotion professionals to locate and time-consuming for them to appraise. Systematic reviews summarize all of the available research evidence on an intervention and should be the first type of research evidence that is looked for. It is also important to understand that having research evidence on the effectiveness, feasibility or acceptability of an intervention is only one piece of the picture. Local needs, funding available and organizational characteristics will also influence whether an intervention is likely to be accepted and successful in promoting health.

References

Deeks JJ, Dinnes J, D'Amico R, Sowden AJ, Sakarovitch C, Song F, Petticrew M, Altman D (2003) Evaluating non-randomised intervention studies. *Health Technology Assessment*, 7(27): 1–186.
Easterbrook PJ, Berlin J, Gopalan R, Matthews DR (1991) Publication bias in clinical research. *Lancet*, 337: 867–72.

Harden A (2001) Finding research evidence: systematic searching, in: Oliver S, Peersman G (eds). Using research for effective health promotion. Buckingham: Open University Press.

Harden A, Peersman G, Oliver S, Oakley A (1999) Identifying primary research on electronic databases to inform decision-making in health promotion: the case of sexual health promotion. *Health Education Journal*, 58: 290–301.

Harden A, Oakley A, Oliver S (2001) Peer-delivered health promotion for young people: a systematic review of different study designs. *Health Education Journal*, 60: 339–53.

Hopewell S, McDonald S, Clarke M, Egger M (2002) Grey literature in meta-analyses of randomized trials of health care interventions. *The Cochrane Database of Methodology Reviews*, 4.

International Committee of Medical Journal Editors (2004) *Uniform Requirements for Manuscripts Submitted to Biomedical Journals: writing and editing for biomedical publication.* Accessed at: http://www.icmje.org/.

Jackson N, Waters E (2005) Guidelines for systematic reviews of health promotion and public health interventions (Version 1.2). Deakin University; Australia.

Kavanagh J, Brunton G, Harden A, Rees R, Oliver S, Oakley A (2002) A method for maximising comprehensiveness in systematic searches and the utility of this approach for the Cochrane Health Promotion and Public Health Field. The 10th Cochrane Colloquium, Stavanger, Norway.

Oliver S, Peersman G (2001) Critical appraisal of research evidence: finding useful and reliable answers, in S. Oliver, G. Peersman (eds) *Using Research for Effective Health Promotion.* Buckingham: Open University Press.

Rotheram-Borus MJ, Cantwell S, Newman PA (2000) HIV prevention programs with heterosexuals. *AIDS*, 14 (supplement 2): 559–67.

Wingood GM, DiClemente RJ (1996) HIV risk reduction interventions for women: a review. *American Journal of Preventive Medicine*, 12(3): 209–17.

SECTION 2

Choosing approaches and methods

4 Cognitive behavioural approaches to health promotion

Overview

The development and maintenance of risk behaviour has its basis in individual and group dynamics, as individuals are strongly influenced by both personal and social factors. The cultural constructions around sex, age, race, ethnicity, physical appearance, socioeconomic status and religion provide strong drivers for how people grow up seeing themselves as an individual and as a member of that culture. While social and group interventions (e.g. peer, media, marketing) in health promotion are covered in later chapters, there are still vital roles that the individual can take in actively appraising and modifying their own health behaviour, either in accordance with, or against, the group norms around them. This chapter explores such individual-based strategies, which are best applied once an individual has decided to change and improve their health-related behaviour. Such strategies are grouped together under the heading cognitive behavioural therapy (CBT) techniques, as they have an emphasis on the identification and modification of people's health-related behaviour and thoughts.

Learning objectives

After reading this chapter, you will be better able to:

- **explain the key features of the cognitive behaviour model**
- **identify key cognitive behavioural therapy issues specific to health behaviour**
- **describe the use of relapse prevention as a specific cognitive behavioural therapy technique in reducing risk behaviour**
- **describe the application of the cognitive behavioural approach to health behaviour using the example of sexual behaviour**

Key terms

Behavioural Observable pattern of human behaviour.

Cognitive Thought processes such as attention, concentration, perception, thinking, learning, memory, beliefs, expectations and assumptions.

Relapse prevention A technique whereby people become aware of the antecedents of their

behaviour and learn to implement behavioural strategies that are incompatible
naviour but still achieve the same function in reducing stress and tension.

The cog.. behavioural model

Over 50 years of research into behavioural and cognitive science has established a
number of core models as to how humans think and act. To a large extent patterns
of both behaviour and thinking (cognition) are learnt during early life, tend to
become habitual once learnt, and continue in that habitual fashion unless a significant external (social or physical) or internal (psychological or biological) event
modifies them. The biopsychosocial model is a template to which CBT is applied. It
encapsulates the three modalities of the biological (physiology, anatomy, bio-
chemistry), psychological (thoughts, feelings, behaviour) and social (relationships,
socioeconomic status, culture and so on) as crucial factors in understanding human
experience. This chapter outlines those internal psychological factors that require
scrutiny and modification before an individual is able to make significant changes
to their health behaviour.

There are a number of key principles in CBT:

1 CBT is robustly evidence-based.
2 The emphasis is on conceptualizing people's presenting problems as formulations and hypotheses which can be tested and adapted across time, rather than
   the use of static diagnoses.
3 The focus is on current factors maintaining the problem, with less attention
   paid towards the aetiology of the problem.
4 Therapy and interventions are problem-based and focused towards finding
   solutions to those problems.
5 Clients/patients are actively involved in their own assessment and treatment.
6 Interventions are aimed at clearly identifiable goals and outcomes, which
   should be measured, monitored and evaluated.

The cognitive behaviour model states that human experience can be broken down
into four factors:

• behaviour (situations, events, actions, skills);
• affect (mood, feelings, emotions);
• cognitions (thoughts, attitudes, beliefs, assumptions, memories, expectations);
• physiology (tension, fitness, diet, health status).

CBT arose from this model as a therapeutic tool to help relieve people from psychological distress. It argues that people become distressed as a consequence of what
behaviour they engage in and, perhaps more importantly, what beliefs they have
about those behaviours. Put simply, behavioural therapy argues that we are what
we do, and cognitive therapy that we are what we think. Therefore, if you
want to change, you need to change what behaviour you engage in, and how you
think about your world and your behaviour. Such changes will then modify how
you feel about yourself, and if the changes in behaviour and cognition are adaptive
and functional to healthy living, then you will feel better about yourself and have a
better quality of life. The relationship between these key factors is outlined in
Figure 4.1.

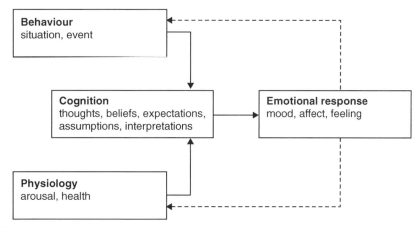

Figure 4.1 A cognitive behavioural model of emotion

The CBT model stipulates that emotions arise not just as a consequence of certain events occurring in our life but also as a consequence of how we think about those events. For example, while a screening procedure for a serious medical condition may seem to be stressful in itself, a person's emotional response to the procedure and to the subsequent test result are also determined by what meaning that procedure and its outcome has for the person. Different expectations as to the level of risk, the perceived seriousness of a positive test result, the expectations of what treatments are available and how effective they are, and the priority that such a condition would have in a person's life all dictate how the person feels about undergoing the procedure. Such an emotional response will then determine how likely the person is to go ahead with the screening behaviour or not. Similarly, a fearful or anxious emotional response then feeds back internally and manifests itself by way of different adrenergic responses such as increased muscle tension, heart rate, sweatiness and so on.

The key concepts in the cognitive and behavioural understanding of health behaviour include:

- Health-related behaviour and cognitions are learned from childhood onwards and, if unchecked, become increasingly habitual.
- People respond to their behaviour being rewarded (positive reinforcement) by increasing that behaviour. They decrease their behaviour if it is followed by an aversive consequence (punishment). They increase behaviour if it is followed by the removal of an unpleasant situation (negative reinforcement) which is often achieved through escaping or avoiding the unpleasant situation.
- The aim of CBT interventions is to identify and break the habitual cycles of unhealthy behaviour and thinking, and to replace these with more adaptive and healthy ones.
- Risk reduction (or harm minimization) techniques have been found to be particularly useful in the reduction of ill health, as these do not aim so much at (often unrealistic) eradication of certain behaviours (intravenous drug use, alcohol use, penetrative sex and so on), but instead aim to minimize the chances

of serious negative health outcomes occurring as a consequence of those behaviours (reduction in needle sharing, control of substance use, barrier methods of contraception and so on).

One mechanism within CBT that helps people understand the determinants of their health behaviour requires that people think about the 'ABC' of that behaviour. The 'A' can stand for 'Activating event' or Antecedent (what actually started the whole thing off?). The 'B' can stand for 'Belief' (what has the person told themselves about that event or behaviour?). The 'C' can stand for the consequences of that behaviour and subsequent cognition (what was the emotional consequence of their thoughts about the event or behaviour, and what did they then go and do about it and what was the consequence of that?).

For example, 'A' could be a demanding environmental situation (such as an argument at work or at home); 'B' could be thoughts along the lines of how awful that argument was and how unacceptable it is to have such arguments; and 'C' could be the person engaging in substance use behaviour (alcohol or some other drug). While the consequence behaviour may be the target of concern (substance use), the CBT model argues that the target behaviour will not be influenced successfully until constructive and adaptive changes are made to the antecedent situation (change work or relationship situation, or change the skills with which the person communicates and problem-solves with other people in these situations and so on), in conjunction with changes in the person's interpretations of such events ('arguments are a normal part of life', 'but what do I need to do to sort this particular problem', and so on).

 Activity 4.1

Try and identify the ABCs of a memorable stressful experience that occurred recently. What was the situation (A); what was your interpretation of that event (B); and what happened as a consequence of it (C)?

 Feedback

When the links are identified between situations, our thoughts about those situations and the consequences of those thoughts, it is possible to understand the powerful manner in which our thoughts influence our response.

Key interventions in CBT

Cognitive behavioural approaches to health-related behaviour include:

* *Monitoring* of target behaviour, in an ongoing manner across many weeks, with an emphasis on identifying the situations which seem to trigger the behaviour, the cognitions, emotions and physiological states associated with those situations, the behaviour the person then engaged in and the subsequent cognitions, emotions and physiological states achieved as a consequence of engaging in the behaviour.

- *Formulations* are developed to help explain the relationships between the situational, cognitive, emotional, physiological and behavioural components in the target behaviour. These formulations can be tested through further monitoring and assessment and can then be modified if required.
- *Goal-setting* is carried out whereby realistic targets are set, that either reduce the harmful outcomes of risk-related behaviour and/or enhance the likelihood of health-seeking behaviour. Graded hierarchies of intermediate goals are then drawn up, so that at any one time the person is only aiming at a target that is slightly higher than what they are already able to achieve, thus giving them more of a chance to experience success in behaviour change.
- *Behavioural skills training* focuses on people identifying skills which could help them resolve the difficult circumstances previously associated with maladaptive health-related behaviours. For example, the person may benefit from being able to communicate better and being more assertive (firm but polite) in difficult situations, or they may benefit from developing their problem-solving skills, or learn how to relax when feeling physically tense (through progressive muscle relaxation, breathing exercises, walking), or find other more constructive ways of engaging in rewarding or stimulating activities.
- *Cognitive restructuring* focuses on people identifying styles of thinking associated with stressful triggers, including the negative, exaggerated self-talk scripts which do not help the person adapt and cope with an otherwise demanding situation. These can be replaced with more constructive self-talk scripts that help the person focus on the task at hand and direct themselves towards behaviour that helps resolve the situation. In general this involves replacing 'I can't' scripts with realistic, achievable 'I can' scripts.
- *Self-instructional training* acknowledges that a person's best behavioural intention can be undermined by particularly acute, demanding situations. Given that high pressure situations can often be predicted in advance, the person is encouraged to generate a script of self-statements that will help focus their attention on the demands of the adaptive behavioural task (communication skills, relaxation, alternative methods of reward and so on) that is incompatible with the health risk behaviour. Such scripts help the person stay on task, and can even be used to help the person manage transgressions from their plan, should they occur. Examples include: 'Stop, focus, concentrate'; 'I knew this could happen, so what do I have to do to get through this?'; 'The tension I am feeling is a cue to begin my coping strategies'; 'think long-term, don't avoid', and so on. Such a strategy is a key component of any performance enhancement psychology.
- *Motivational interviewing* is aimed at helping shift people from a state where they are not interested in any behaviour change. This technique is covered in much more detail in Chapter 5.
- *Relapse prevention* (RP) enables people to implement their intentions to change their behaviour, once they are clearly motivated to do so. It does this through detailed monitoring and identification of the behavioural, cognitive, emotional and physiological antecedents that precede specific risk behaviour, and the compilation and activation of an alternative behavioural response that can be initiated prior to the risk behaviour occurring. This technique is outlined in more detail below.

Activity 4.2

> Monitor an important/interesting aspect of your behaviour using a diary, for a one-week period. Identify the circumstances that may be related to its occurrence: day of the week, time of day, what were you doing just before/after the behaviour, what were you feeling like before/after, what kinds of things you were thinking about before/after, how strong/severe was the actual behaviour and how long did it last for.

 Feedback

> After recording such aspects of behaviour over many days, patterns begin to emerge that indicate the habitual manner in which certain behaviours occur only under certain circumstances, which are in turn interpreted in characteristic ways by the individual. The response can have certain rewarding (often short-term) consequences for the person.

RP – the development of CBT strategies to reduce habitual risk behaviours

RP was initially developed by Marlatt and Gordon and others as a CBT strategy to help people with their alcohol dependency (e.g. Marlatt and Gordon 1985). Following its success in alcohol abuse it was adapted for a range of other risk behaviours, including smoking and drug use.

RP was developed as an alternative to the abstinence treatment model for 'alcoholism'. The abstinence model conceptualizes alcohol dependency as a biologically determined illness that the 'alcoholic' had no control over, which requires external pharmacological and spiritual interventions to treat, but which the person is never free from. Indeed, there is growing evidence that genetics play an important interactive role in 'alcoholism', and the Alcoholics Anonymous model has undoubtedly been a major factor in helping many people eliminate 'addictive' behaviours.

However, a CBT-based formulation of habitual behaviours stresses the use of alcohol as a maladaptive avoidant/escape coping strategy applied by people who lack more adaptive coping strategies in the face of stressful life events. A lapse or relapse back into binge drinking is seen as a consequence of a whole series of psychological events that occur across time, and control over that drinking behaviour can only be achieved through the identification of the interrelated antecedent events preceding the relapse and the implementation of alternative, more adaptive strategies for responding to the high-risk situations associated with the cumulative stressors. RP emphasizes the development of an individual's own ability to understand and control their behaviour, and it accommodates relapses back into risk behaviour as momentary lapses that do not need to continue.

Key issues in RP

Mapping the behavioural, cognitive, emotional and physiological antecedents to risk behaviour

The application of RP techniques requires that the person understands the mechanism by which their risk behaviour comes about, and what it is in response to. To do this, they need to monitor their target behaviour closely, collecting information on the exact time and place that the target behaviour occurs, and then back-tracking to identify the flow of behavioural, cognitive, physiological and emotional events that occurred for the few hours (and sometimes days) prior to the onset of the risk behaviour. This can be done retrospectively, but it may be more exact to do it prospectively, through the use of diaries which monitor these factors daily. Of particular importance is the build-up of aversive behavioural events (aggression, agitation, conflict, isolation, overcrowding, multiple tasking and so on), negative cognitions (not achieving, disapproval, lack of control, helplessness, aversive expectation, sense of injustice and so on), heightened physiological arousal/tension (tension headache, increased heart/breathing rate, muscle tension in stomach, back, jaw and so on), and distressing emotions (anger, anxiety, fear, depression and so on), the combination of which can trigger a build-up of stress and distress that will require the application of some form of adaptive/maladaptive stress management behaviour to reduce. An outline of such a flow is provided in Figure 4.2; each box may be minutes or hours (or even days) apart from the next box in the sequence.

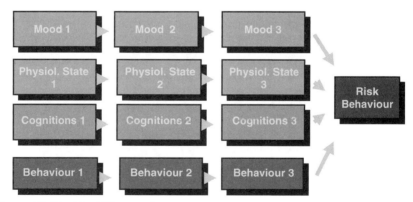

Figure 4.2 Combined RP antecedents

Once the person has done this type of monitoring for a few weeks, clear patterns of health-related behaviour and its antecedents usually emerge, along with an appreciation of the short-term benefits of responding to those situations with their habitual risk behaviour (which often achieves relief through avoidance/escape), and an appreciation of the long-term harmful consequences of continuing to engage in that particular behaviour.

Identifying high-risk situations

Monitoring behaviour invariably results in people being able to identify the build-up that precedes the onset of significant risk behaviour. With this insight comes the realization that should such a profile occur again they must acknowledge that they are entering a high-risk situation (HRS) that, if unchecked, will be highly likely to result in the onset of habitual risk behaviour. HRSs become particularly relevant once the person has placed themselves in a situation where they are much more able to engage in the risk behaviour. For example, such HRSs can include a person entering a venue that provides, or otherwise enables them to obtain alcohol, cigarettes or other drugs; obtaining junk food from the shops; going to venues where sexual partners can be found without taking any condoms with them; taking a vehicle to a place where alcohol is available and drinking encouraged; and so on. People are then in a position to know that, if a specific profile of aversive psychological events has occurred, and they then move towards setting up the risk behaviour, then they are entering an HRS which will greatly increase the chance of them engaging in the risk behaviour. The development of such HRSs should then be associated with a clear warning signal to the person that they need to be careful in the immediate future.

Recognizing seemingly innocent choices

People can often find themselves stringing together behaviours which, in isolation, seem innocent and benign, but which, when strung together, result in the person finding themselves in the middle of an HRS, seemingly unprepared. Such seemingly innocent choices (SICs; sometimes referred to as apparently irrelevant decisions or AIDs) can be illustrated by the following example:

> A man has controlled his drinking for some time, but has had a bad few days with stress at work. It's the weekend, and he has just had an argument with his wife at home and is feeling tense and agitated. He wants to calm his nerves by having a cigarette, but has run out, so needs to go down to the shop to get some. He chooses the shop next to the pub, although he has no intention of going in to the pub or drinking. He buys his cigarettes but finds he needs a cigarette lighter; unfortunately, the shop is out of lighters but the off licence attached to the pub has lighters, so he goes to buy one. While he's there, an old drinking buddy calls out to him from the bar, so he agrees to go through and have a soft drink and a brief chat. He arrives home five hours later, very drunk.

In this example, the man may well be making genuine decisions that are not at all related to an intention to binge drink. In another situation where he was not already feeling agitated and distressed, he may well have been able to go down the HRS path and pull out before binge drinking. But when all these variables are set in combination, HRSs and chained SICs will greatly increase the probability of a lapse, and it is a goal in RP for people to identify this and be very aware of when it is happening. It is otherwise very easy for people to distort, deny and rationalize these SICs, such that they seem more benign.

Identifying rewarding dimensions to risk behaviour

People engage in behaviour for good reasons, as outlined earlier. It is therefore vital that people identify and understand the powerful rewarding effect that their risk behaviour has on their lives. Most risk behaviour helps people feel good, but it is most problematic when its effect is to stop them feeling bad (negative reinforcement). Thus, the rewarding properties of some risk behaviour (e.g. binge eating, binge drinking, drug dependency, unsafe sex, failure to attend health screening procedures and even failure to attend vaccination programmes) can all be understood in terms of short-term avoidant/escape of aversive experiences, via the removal of a distressing psychological state (through nurturing or sensation-seeking behaviour, or via the avoidance of painful or anxiety-inducing medical procedures). RP identifies the role of selective attention towards these positive expectancies, some of which have, at one level, strong socially enhancing properties such as the social enjoyment and confidence inspiring nature of drinking or drug-taking with friends.

Identifying alternative functional strategies to HRSs

Once people understand the rewarding properties of their risk behaviour, they are in a much better position to comprehend the need to provide alternative strategies to help manage difficult situations and the need for these alternatives to be at least as powerful as their risk behaviours in helping them feel good, as opposed to stopping them feel bad.

In the case of comforting or sensation-seeking behaviour, people need to identify and become proficient in applying more adaptive coping strategies for the difficulties they have in life. These invariably involve more learning and better use of communication, problem-solving and decision-making skills, along with goal-setting, time management, conflict resolution and relaxation skills.

In the case of avoidant behaviour around medical procedures, people need to learn that the short-term benefits of avoiding stressful procedures are far outweighed by both the long-term stress and uncertainty of not being screened or vaccinated, and the long-term costs of not addressing treatable conditions early enough. Often this can be achieved through the use of a 3 × 2 decision-making matrix; along the top are two columns such as 'Test' and 'Don't test', and down the side are three rows, 'six days', 'six months' and 'six years'. People are then encouraged to think through the psychological, social and medical consequences of each cell in the matrix.

Activity 4.3

Draw up a decision matrix for a behaviour you have been avoiding, and think through the short-, medium- and long-term consequences of engaging versus not engaging in the behaviour. When you have mapped these out, what decision should you make that will have the best outcome in six years time?

Feedback

It is invariably the case that six years of worry far exceeds the avoidance of six days of worry.

Managing the abstinence violation effect for lapses

The RP model conceptualizes lapses as a momentary mistake that the person can learn from, refrain from, and limit themselves to. This is in contrast to the abstinence model of substance misuse, which implies that if people engage in risk behaviour after a period of abstinence, then they have failed and lost all control of their behaviour, and this is often associated with an immediate exacerbation of the behaviour (including a binge). RP sets up management of lapses in advance, encourages the person to reapply a controlled limit on their behaviour, and trains them to apply cognitive restructuring skills to minimize the adverse effects of abstinence violation.

Multifactorial skills

RP stresses the need for people to make changes in a number of other areas that are more or less directly associated with the problem behaviour. These include education around risk behaviours and stress management, re-engaging in activities previously found rewarding (recreational pursuits, sports, hobbies) and changes in overall lifestyle.

Efficacy of RP in changing health behaviour

More detailed overviews of the RP model are provided elsewhere (e.g. Larimer *et al.* 1999), as are overviews of its efficacy in changing health behaviour (e.g., Irvin *et al.* 1999). In summary, meta-analyses indicate that RP is effective at improving health behaviour, and is most effective in alcohol dependency and multiple drug use, especially when used in conjunction with other strategies, including global lifestyle changes and stress management techniques. RP may not be any more effective in producing short-term reductions in some habitual behaviour compared to some other techniques. However, RP is most effective in reducing the frequency and severity of relapses, and in helping people recover from relapses, especially in the long term, in much the same way that CBT has been shown to be most effective in reducing long-term recurrences in depressed mood and anxiety.

RP has been applied and evaluated in a range of settings incorporating multi-factorial intervention strategies, including smoking, offending behaviour, violence, unsafe sex and psychiatric readmissions. Unfortunately, given that RP was only one part of the intervention package applied in these settings, it has not been possible to isolate and quantify the influence that the RP component contributed to any treatment effects. Nonetheless, its validity is often cited as a key component to many programmes aimed at changing behaviour.

Theoretical social-cognitive models of individual health behaviour

Health psychologists have adapted CBT models and generic social behaviour models to specific health-related behaviour for a number of decades now. Of particular relevance are (1) the Health Belief Model (HBM: Becker 1974), which highlighted the role of individual perceptions of cost/benefit and ability/barriers to the health behaviour; and (2) the theory of reasoned action (TRA: Ajzen and Fishbein 1980) which highlighted the dominant explanatory and predictive power of an individual's perception of their peer group norms relating to a class of behaviours and the desire for the individual to adhere to those perceived norms. Subsequent work on these and other models has increasingly highlighted the impact that social normative behaviour has on the health behaviour of an individual, although critics still argue that these models fail to fully incorporate and quantify group and social processes in the prediction of individual health behaviour. Clear examples of this in relation to health behaviour include the power of peers, media, music and entertainment in determining adolescent and young adult substance use and sexual behaviour.

Application of CBT strategies in health promotion: the example of sexual risk behaviour

An example of a more contemporary health behaviour model that attempts to better accommodate social normative factors into the understanding of an individual's health-related behaviour is Fisher and Fisher's (1992) information-motivation-behaviour model (IMB) of sexual behaviour. This model argues that there are three key determinants of sexual risk behaviour. (1) *information*: the degree to which the individual is informed about sex, sexually transmitted infections (STIs), and the prevention of STIs; (2) *behavioural skills*: the degree to which the individual is able to implement safer sex strategies (ability to obtain and use condoms, negotiate condom use with reluctant partners, access sexual health services and so on); and (3) *motivation*: the individual's attitude towards safer sex (perceived risk, self-efficacy, perceived group norms regarding condom use, intentions to use condoms and so on).

Subsequent research into the IMB models has confirmed the dominant role that motivational factors play in the prediction of sexual behaviour (Fisher and Fisher 2000). While optimal levels of information are essential in enabling people to make informed decisions about their sexual health, once these optimal levels are reached the provision of additional information does little to add to the prediction of sexual behaviour. In this regard, the provision of basic sex education and information around STIs and the prevention of STIs is crucial for groups who lack that information; however, the costly provision of further sexual health promotion materials through expensive poster, leaflet and media campaigns may well not be a good use of prevention funds if targeted at people who are already well informed. It's one thing for people to know what to do, but something completely different for them to have the ability to behaviourally implement that knowledge; interventions aimed at enhancing people's safer sex skills are more effective in changing behaviour once an optimal level of knowledge and information has been achieved. But the most important factor is a person's motivation to implement safer sex strategies. People may well know it all and even be able to do it, but if they don't think it relates to them (low perceived risk), or have other more important priorities (including basic needs like shelter and food, money or immediate gratification), or feel they will be ridiculed if they do something that is seen by others as unnecessary or 'uncool', then they will not engage in any behaviour change. Such motivational factors have been found to be by far the strongest predictors of sexual behaviour change in many populations, and are therefore a major barrier in the implementation of any sexual health promotion programme.

The process of developing programmes based on frameworks such as the IMB model is firstly to do an assessment of where an individual's (or group's) strengths and deficits lie. What is the level of awareness and knowledge around HIV and STIs? What is the level of efficacy and ability to carry out the behaviours required to implement the safer sex strategy? What are the attitudes towards safer sexual behaviour and hence what is the level of motivation to change/consolidate? Once the person (or group's) deficit profile is identified, interventions aimed at reducing the deficits need to be implemented. If there is an information deficit, then factual information about HIV/STI transmission and prevention needs to be provided along with the correction of common misconceptions regarding HIV/STIs. If there is a skill deficit, then skills training needs to be conducted around condom acquisition and use, abstinence, communication skills, accessing sexual health services and relapse prevention. If there is a motivational deficit, then attitudinal change work needs to be carried out using motivational interviewing, peer discussion/ videos, and cognitive restructuring and self-instruction. The final stage of any intervention is to do a follow-up assessment of changes in knowledge, attitudes and behaviour, to ascertain the effectiveness of the intervention. Nothing can be assumed about the attitudes and behaviour of any individual or group; baseline and follow-up assessments must always be carried out to inform any particular intervention.

Summary

There is an established evidence base for the application of CBT techniques in the promotion of a broad range of people's health-related behaviour. The detailed monitoring of habitual cognitive, physiological, emotional and behavioural factors associated with any target health behaviour helps people understand the function that these behaviours have, and lends itself towards a comprehensive intervention programme aimed at modifying and controlling the antecedents and consequences of the target behaviour. People's dysfunctional behaviour often occurs in response to their desire to avoid or escape distressing situations. CBT therefore encourages people to make changes in their behaviour and in the way they think about their behaviour so they can better cope with the distressing situation without resorting to short-term avoidant strategies.

RP is a specific cognitive behavioural technique which helps identify the chain of cognitive, behavioural, emotional and physiological events which habitually precede problem behaviours. This enables the person to identify the warning signs of future slides towards that problem behaviour, and helps direct them towards more adaptive alternative strategies to cope with the stressful situations. People's attitudes about and motivations towards health behaviour are strong predictors of health behaviour, above and beyond their level of knowledge about or ability to perform protective behaviours, and it is for this reason that attention must also be paid towards factors which influence those attitudes, including peer and social group norms.

References

Ajzen I (1991) The theory of planned behaviour. *Organizational Behavior and Human Decision Processes*, 50: 179–211.

Ajzen I, Fishbein M (1980) *Understanding Attitudes and Predicting Social Behavior*. Englewood Cliffs, NJ: Prentice-Hall.

Becker MH (1974) The health belief model and personal health behavior. *Health Education Monographs* 2(4).

Fisher JD, Fisher WA (1992) Changing AIDS risk behaviour. *Psychological Bulletin*, 111: 455–75.

Fisher JD, Fisher WA (2000) Theoretical approaches to individual-level change in HIV risk behaviour, in J Peterson, R DiClemente (eds) *Handbook of HIV Prevention*. New York: Plenum Press.

Irvin JE, Bowers CA, Dunn ME, Wang MC (1999) Efficacy of relapse prevention: a meta-analytic review. *Journal of Consulting and Clinical Psychology*, 67(4): 563–70.

Larimer ME, Palmer RS, Marlett GA (1999) Relapse prevention: an overview of Marlatt's cognitive behavioural model. *Alcohol Research and Health*, 23(2): 151–60.

Marlatt GA and Gordon JR (1985) *Relapse Prevention: Maintenance Strategies in the Treatment of Addictive Behaviours*. New York: Brunner/Mazel.

Further reading

Fisher WA, Fisher JD, Harmen J (2003) The information-motivational-behavioural skills model: a general psychological approach to understanding and promoting health behaviour, in J. Suls, KA Wallston (eds) *Social Psychological Foundations of Health and Illness*. Oxford: Blackwell.

5 | Motivational interviewing in health promotion

Overview

One of the five action areas for health promotion, described in the Ottawa Charter, is the development of personal skills. Developing personal skills aims to give people greater control over their health and the environments in which they live. Such work often takes place via face-to-face interactions with health professionals, voluntary health workers and community workers. The settings for such interventions include hospitals, primary care clinics, schools, workplaces, community settings and the home. How a face-to-face intervention is conducted (the process) is as important as what is intended to be achieved (the outcome). In this chapter, you will learn about one approach for communicating with people during face-to-face interventions called motivational interviewing (MI). You will look at its development and the key concepts and principles underlying it. You will also explore its application to different health behaviours and consider its efficacy.

Learning objectives

After reading this chapter, you will be better able to:

- **describe the key concepts and principles underlying motivational interviewing**
- **describe the differences between motivational interviewing and more traditional approaches to behaviour change**
- **discuss the relative strengths and limitations of motivational interviewing**
- **describe the efficacy of motivational interviewing for different health behaviours**
- **explain when motivational interviewing might be used alone and when in concert with other approaches**

Key terms

Ambivalence A conflict between two courses of action each of which has perceived costs and benefits associated with it. The exploration and resolution of ambivalence is a key feature in motivational interviewing.

Change talk Involves a client expressing personal advantages of changing behaviour, optimism for change, intention to change and the disadvantages of no change or the status quo.

Motivation Incentives or driving forces that encourage the adoption of health-promoting behaviours or lifestyles.

> **Motivational interviewing (MI)** A client-centred, directive method for enhancing intrinsic motivation to change by exploring and resolving ambivalence.
>
> **Readiness** Used in motivational interviewing to refer to the degree to which a client is resolved to change their lifestyle or behaviour.
>
> **Resistance** Opposition to changing behaviour, often expressed as a series of 'excuses' for not wanting or needing to change.
>
> **Transtheoretical model** Developed to describe and explain the different stages in behaviour change. The model is based on the premise that behaviour change is a process, not an event, and that individuals have different levels of motivation or readiness to change.

The development of a new approach

MI was developed in the addictions field by specialist alcohol workers seeking a different approach to consultations that frequently led to disagreement about the extent to which a client's drinking represented a problem. It was first described by William Miller who subsequently defined it as a 'client-centred, directive method for enhancing intrinsic motivation to change by exploring and resolving ambivalence' (Miller and Rollnick 2002). As suggested by this definition, the central tenet of the approach is the exploration and resolution of ambivalence. As defined above, ambivalence involves conflict between two courses of action each of which has perceived costs and benefits associated with it. In MI, the practitioner's task is to facilitate expression of both sides of the ambivalence and guide the client towards an acceptable resolution that increases the probability of change and decreases the probability of the status quo.

The focus on the exploration and resolution of ambivalence distinguishes MI from more traditional approaches to health behaviour change which are based on a 'medical model' or disease-centred approach. The disease-centred approach is characterized by the practitioner extracting information about the presenting 'problem' that will enable some form of diagnosis or behavioural assessment. This is followed by the 'prescription' of a strategy for resolving the problem as seen from the practitioner's perspective. In individual-level health promotion, it is common to collect information on a given behaviour in order to determine whether it presents a health risk. If the behaviour is deemed to be 'risky' by the practitioner, he or she is likely to counsel the person on the health risks of persisting with the behaviour, and/or the benefits of changing that behaviour, along with advice on how best to change. Implicit in this approach is that health is a primary motivating force for change and if people have the correct knowledge, attitude and skills then they will adopt more health-promoting behaviours.

There is a wealth of evidence to show the approach described above does not reflect reality. Persuasion to adopt a particular health behaviour can often be met with resistance, displayed as a series of 'excuses' for not wanting or needing to change. Resistance to change is usually countered by attempts to further persuade or coerce the person into change by using logic to change maladaptive or irrational beliefs, or offering strategies to cope with obstacles to change (Miller and Rollnick 1991). The disease-centred approach is not a malicious attempt to force people to change their behaviour but stems from a genuine desire to help resolve people's health problems, many of which will be significantly influenced by their lifestyle. It reflects traditional teaching methods in medical schools that place emphasis on an accurate and precise diagnosis of the presenting condition. Such an approach is less appropriate in individual health promotion encounters where the focus is on health behaviours, many of which are not purely under volitional control.

MI presents an alternative approach which is more in keeping with modern thinking on patient-led medical encounters. There are parallels between MI and the client-centred therapy of Carl Rogers (1957) where there is greater emphasis on understanding the client's perspective. During MI, clients are actively encouraged to express their own reasons for and against change, how consistent their current behaviour is with the achievement of their life goals or core values, and what if any behaviour change will be pursued. This is not to say MI never includes health promotion advice or information about ways to deal with obstacles to change; rather it is a matter of timing. When ambivalence is resolved and there is a strong commitment and intention to change, MI practitioners may incorporate behaviour-change strategies such as self-monitoring, goal-setting and reinforcement, with the client's permission.

 Activity 5.1

A person with a chronic cough is consulting a doctor. The doctor knows the person has smoked for many years and believes the cough is a direct result of the smoking. Consider the following two scenarios and what the smoker's responses might be to each, and which one is more likely to lead to exploration of ambivalence.

1   The doctor says, 'I know we've discussed this many times before, but we really do need to find a way to get you to stop smoking. Your cough is only going to get much worse and is likely to lead to something much more serious. I can help you to stop, either by prescribing some nicotine replacement therapy or referring you to the smoking cessation nurse. What do you think?'

2   The doctor says, 'As we've discussed before, I believe your cough is related to your smoking. I wonder on a scale from 0–10 how motivated are you right now to stop smoking?' 0 on the scale is not motivated at all and 10 is very motivated. The person gives a score between 0–10. The doctor asks why the score is not a lower number and listens to the patient's response. The doctor asks, 'What would have to change for you to give a higher number, feel more motivated?'

 Feedback

1   The doctor tries to persuade the person to quit smoking by trying to heighten the person's perceived risk of smoking and suggested a course of action. This ignores the person's perspective entirely. If, as is likely, the person feels ambivalent about smoking, they will not only perceive the costs of smoking, but also the personal costs of quitting and the benefits of continuing. The doctor's focus on just one part of the person's ambivalence is likely to focus the person's mind onto other parts of their ambivalence,

which they will express verbally. So a typical response might be, 'Yes, but I find smoking is the only way I can cope with the stress in my life.' This type of dialogue will often result in the doctor making the case for change and the smoker making the case for no change.

2 This strategy is designed immediately to encourage the smoker to express all aspects of their ambivalence without any judgement from the doctor.

Motivation for change

Motivation is often described as a necessary ingredient in achieving behaviour change and yet is seldom defined. Where it is defined, it is common for motivation to be regarded as part of an individual's personality or character (Miller and Rollnick 1991). Such a definition can lead to failure to change behaviour being attributed to a 'lack' of motivation on the part of the client. In MI, motivation is seen more as a product of interpersonal process and one of the most important aspects of health-behaviour consultations. A pragmatic translation of the term motivation is that it represents a behavioural probability. When it is high, the likelihood of behaviour change increases and vice versa. Consequently, any aspect of a health care encounter that increases the probability of change can be regarded as motivational. In MI, this means trying to identify the key elements of the interpersonal process that lead to change. Three necessary components of motivation have been described as:

- readiness to change;
- the importance or value placed on change;
- confidence in the ability to change.

Put simply, if a person thinks change will lead to valued outcomes, they are confident they can achieve change, and there are no competing priorities, then motivation will be high.

Principles of MI

There are four general principles that underpin MI practice: express empathy; develop a discrepancy; roll with resistance; and support self-efficacy (Miller and Rollnick 2002). *Expressing empathy* or showing acceptance of the client's perspective and feelings is a key attribute of the MI practitioner. This is achieved through skilful reflective listening. This means that a client's ambivalence about change is seen as understandable, normal and valid. Change can be motivated by *developing a discrepancy* between present behaviour and important personal goals or how one would like to be, within the empathic style. A goal of MI is to evoke this discrepancy from within the person and amplify it.

In health behaviour consultations, it is common for clients to be unforthcoming about changing behaviour, even when it appears obvious to the practitioner that change would significantly benefit the client's health. Attempts to persuade or coerce a client towards change when they are not ready are likely to be met with resistance. The third principle of MI is to be able to *roll with resistance* rather than confronting it. Resistance is often provoked when the practitioner misjudges the importance a client places on health, how confident they are about change or how ready they are to change. Resistance will also be encountered if the client feels that their freedom to choose what to do is being challenged. In MI, resistance usually results from the practitioner doing the wrong thing at the wrong time and signals a need to do something different (Miller and Rollnick 2002).

The greater the belief a person has in their ability to change, the greater the probability that they will (Bandura 2004). *Supporting self-efficacy* is the fourth principle of MI and seeks to encourage the client that change is possible by exploring the successes of others and showing a willingness to support the client through change. In addition, the practitioner's belief in the client's capacity for change also leads to greater confidence in the client.

Aside from the general goal of exploring and resolving ambivalence, a key strategy in MI is eliciting *change talk*. Change talk involves the client expressing personal advantages of changing behaviour, optimism for change, intention to change and the disadvantages of no change or the status quo. It is based on the theory that people are more likely to accept and act on what they hear themselves say rather than what others say (see the next section on MI's theoretical basis). The more clients defend a position, the more they become committed to it. Engaging in change talk during a consultation means reduced resistance or commitment to the status quo.

 Activity 5.2

What follows is an extract of an MI session talking about physical activity. Read through the transcript and answer the following questions.

1   Who is doing most of the talking, the practitioner (P) or the client (C)?
2   How many change talk statements are there from the client?
3   How many reflective listening statements are there from the practitioner?
4   How does the client express a discrepancy between what they say is important in their life and their current behaviour?

C: I've just spent two days walking in the Brecons [a mountain range in Wales] because I like to walk. I think if I lived in Wales I'd exercise every day, but where I live, there are no nice hills, just roundabouts. At the moment I feel like I want to keep going because it felt so good. I have a sense of well-being when I've exercised. I always say that when I get back, I'm going to keep this up but of course I don't, I just get back into my old routine.

P: So you've noticed that when you do some exercise there's something quite pleasurable about it.

C: Oh yes, I mean I do like to swim. There was a point in my life, after I'd had children, when I thought I must do some exercise and I went swimming for six months. It does feel good, but it's the motivation, getting myself motivated to go and do it.

P: But when you do find the motivation, you've actually found it beneficial.

C: It sounds silly but I do want to exercise, I do want to do it. I see these adverts in the local paper for cheap membership at the local gym but I worry what the people might be like.

P: You worry that you might not fit in.

C: Yes, if I had someone to go with, or pull me down there, I would go. When I did go swimming I had more energy and felt less tired. Talking like this makes me think why aren't I doing it? But it's the motivation.

P: So you have experienced a number of benefits of being more active but there's still something getting in your way.

C: Yes, I was even a lower weight when I exercised more. Now I'm a stone heavier than I used to be.

P: You've noticed that how much exercise you do is linked to your weight.

C: Yes, even after a week's walking holiday last year I lost weight and felt so much better.

 Feedback

What this extract shows is that when MI is going well, the client will be doing most of the talking, they will frequently engage in change talk and the practitioner will mainly respond to the client with reflective listening statements. In this extract the client expresses a discrepancy by displaying a degree of confusion when they reflect on the fact they keep stating that physical activity is good for them yet they aren't doing it.

Theoretical basis

MI is not a new theory of behaviour change but an interpersonal style that draws on a number of existing psychosocial theories of behaviour change (e.g. Bandura 2004) as well as the work of Rogers (1957). To simplify, the psychosocial theories hypothesize that behaviour change is more likely when:

- the perceived benefits of change outweigh the perceived costs;
- change will lead to social approval, not disapproval;
- change will lead to self-satisfaction and is consistent with highly valued, broader life goals;
- desirable outcomes are within one's personal control and are achievable through one's own actions;
- they are few obstacles or barriers to achieving change;
- opportunities for change are high.

MI acknowledges that people will vary in how ready they are to change and that the level of readiness should be taken into account during an intervention. This is consistent with an influential model of behaviour change, called the *trans-theoretical model*, which theorizes that people move through a series of stages as they change behaviour. The model emphasizes the importance of matching the correct intervention to each stage of readiness to change (Prochaska *et al.* 1992). The transtheoretical model describes time periods for some stages, indicating a degree of stability, whereas in MI readiness is regarded as a more continuous phenomena in a constant state of flux (Resnicow *et al.* 2002). As well as drawing on the ideas of Prochaska *et al.*, MI also draws on self-perception theory (Bem 1972), which posits that people become more committed to that which they hear themselves argue for and defend.

Rather than having one underlying theory, MI has been described as having a 'spirit' that underlies it (Miller and Rollnick 2002). The 'spirit' of MI is captured in three fundamental approaches to a consultation. First, the relationship between a practitioner and client is collaboration, rather than an authoritarian one. Second, evoking intrinsic motivation for change is more desirable than trying to impose it from without. Third, the practitioner respects the client's autonomy and acknowledges that responsibility for change lies with the client. The spirit of MI is reminiscent of the 'conditions for change' in client-centred therapy described by Rogers (1957), which proposed that a therapeutic alliance and practitioner empathy are necessary for change. These conditions for change plus the directive method of selectively reinforcing change talk and 'commitment language' go some way to forming a theoretical basis for MI.

Adaptations of MI

Since its inception in the drug and alcohol field, there has been considerable interest in adapting MI for other health behaviours, particularly those associated with chronic conditions, such as cardiovascular and metabolic diseases. This is probably due to health promotion workers confronting issues of adherence and motivation similar to those faced by drug and alcohol workers. MI and various adaptations of it have subsequently been applied to smoking, diet, physical activity, water purification, treatment compliance and gambling. As noted above, MI was originally developed for specialist settings and highly trained addictions counsellors, where it is common for there to be multiple sessions of significant duration. In contrast, health promotion practitioners are often restricted by the number of sessions at their disposal and the duration of each session. It is not uncommon to have just one brief encounter with a person. Inevitably, this has meant that derivatives of MI as it was originally described have been developed either through trial and error or intentionally, based on research and clinical practice (Emmons and Rollnick 2001). To reflect the differences between MI and its more 'dilute' derivatives, based on its spirit and principles, two alternative kinds of behaviour change intervention have been described (Miller and Rollnick 2002):

- *Brief advice* (BA) is appropriate for short interventions lasting 5–15 minutes, where health promotion is likely to be opportunistic rather than sought. The primary goal of this type of intervention, particularly if the person is not ready to change, is to initiate thinking about changing behaviour. Information is likely to be exchanged and the encounter is likely to be more directive than MI with less focus on choice and personal responsibility for change.
- *Behaviour change counselling* (BCC) requires more time, up to 30 minutes, and can take place in an opportunistic or help-seeking setting. It has a greater focus

on identifying client goals and building motivation for change than does BA. Strategies adopted are more likely to be based on readiness to change and the practitioner will have received more training and be more skilled in expressing empathy than the practitioner delivering BA alone.

By contrast, MI often takes place for an hour at a time, mostly with help-seeking clients. There is a much greater emphasis on resolving ambivalence and creating a discrepancy. The practitioner style is very much empathic and he or she is highly skilled in reflective listening and eliciting change talk.

One important reason for the distinction between BA, BCC and MI is in interpreting research findings. It is quite common for people to refer to an intervention as MI because it is loosely based on MI principles. If the 'adapted' method is subject to a trial of its efficacy and no change in behaviour is seen, it is likely to be attributed to the ineffectiveness of MI. Closer inspection of the adaptations may reveal that the intervention had little in common with the parent method apart from a desire to elicit motivation in a non-confrontational style. Some adaptations will be necessary depending on the setting and the behaviour being discussed. In addictive behaviours, people are more likely to be seeking help and resistance will be more intense than, say, someone considering increasing their intake of fruit and vegetables. Change in addictive behaviours sometimes involves abstinence, whereas non-addictive behaviours normally require modifying existing behaviours. It might appear that the focus in addictive behaviours is more on the 'to-be-lost' behaviour rather than on the challenge of adopting a new behaviour. However, this is not always the case. For example, when trying to incorporate more physical activity into one's life, time has to be freed from some other aspect of the lifestyle, such as time for family or relaxation. The person may place great value on these behaviours and be reluctant to reduce time spent on them. Modifying health behaviours often requires short-term discomfort for future benefit in people who don't perceive they have a problem.

The various differences in the adaptations to MI raises important issues about evaluation. Integrated analysis of the findings of formative and process evaluation along with outcome data can help identify the specific effects of the components of MI. When reviewing studies of MI, it is important to ask: what was the specific method being examined?; how competent were the practitioners in the method?; and how well was the method adhered to? (Miller and Rollnick 2002). Only a few studies, which state they are evaluating MI, provide data on formative and process evaluation (Tappin et al. 2005). This is an important consideration for future studies.

Activity 5.3

Read the extracts of the methods sections from the following two studies. Think about the amount of detail provided about the intervention in each study and attempt to identify whether study participants received BA, BCC or MI. How confident are you that the integrity of the approach was upheld and why?

Study one

All participants received their baseline results (blood pressure, weight for height, activity level, aerobic capacity, smoking and alcohol consumption) and a pack containing information on the benefits of physical activity, other lifestyle factors (smoking, alcohol, weight and diet), recommended activity levels for men and women of different ages [as well as] 19 leaflets on leisure facilities and activities available locally. Brief advice was given, comparing individual's results with recommended levels and highlighting details in the information pack. Those in the control group received no further intervention.

Participants randomised to receive brief intervention (interventions 1 and 2) were offered one motivational interview within two weeks of their baseline assessment. Those receiving intervention 2 [also] received 30 vouchers at the interview. Participants randomised to receive intensive intervention (interventions 3 and 4) were offered six motivational interviews over 12 weeks, the first within two weeks of the baseline assessment. Those in intervention 4 also received 30 vouchers at the first interview.

Motivational interviewing is a technique for negotiating behaviour change that uses the stages of change model of behaviour change. A health visitor, who was trained in motivational interviewing, delivered the motivational interviews. Interviews were scheduled to last 40 minutes and took place at the practice or local leisure centre. They aimed to promote safe, effective physical activity but did not prescribe particular activities. A structured record was completed at each interview, a copy of which was given to participants; this was used to review progress for those attending more than one interview (Harland et al. 1999).

Study two

Motivational interviewing is a one to one counselling style designed for treating addictions. Its 'stages of change' model is widely taught on smoking cessation training courses but may not apply during pregnancy. We used a randomised controlled trial to determine whether the quit rate for pregnant smokers increases with motivational interviewing provided at home by specially trained midwives. A consultant provided five days of training in motivational interviewing followed by one day a month throughout the study, using midwives' own recorded interviews to focus development of skills. Midwives provided standard health promotion including information on smoking and pregnancy from a health education book given to all pregnant women in Scotland. Women in the intervention group were offered two to five additional home visits of about 30 minutes' duration from the same study midwife. Midwives made six attempts to contact women, including the home visit arranged at enrolment, two to three telephone calls, one or two 'cold' calls to the house, and sending a letter asking them to telephone a free number.

All 625 home visits were recorded and stored as digital files. A 10% (n = 63) random sample of interviews was transcribed and sent to the Center for Alcoholism Substance Abuse and Addictions, University of New Mexico for content analysis using the motivational interviewing skills code (Tappin et al. 2005).

 Feedback

In the first study very little information is provided on what the health visitor did during the consultations or how much of what was done actually reflected textbook descriptions of MI. Furthermore, there is no indication of how proficient the health visitor was in delivering MI. The absence of detail on what study participants received prevents us from determining if MI or any derivative of it was actually being examined in this study. Therefore, it is possible that what participants actually received was not MI or one of its derivatives at all. The results of the study indicated no difference in self-reported physical activity between groups. Without more detail about exactly what participants were exposed to, it is not possible to determine if the lack of effect was due to MI not working or the intervention not actually involving MI.

The second study provides a little more detail about MI and the amount of training the midwives received. Specifically, all interventions were recorded and transcribed. A random sample was then independently assessed for MI integrity using validated assessment instruments. This level of quality control allows us to be confident that the intervention was delivered as intended and that high quality MI was delivered. What these two extracts highlight is the difficulty of ascertaining whether or not the exposure variable in the study was actually MI or not. Future studies need to consider what is actually being evaluated: is it the effectiveness of MI on changing client health behaviour or the effectiveness of training to change practitioner behaviour?

Training of practitioners

MI is intuitively appealing to practitioners as it relieves them of the responsibility for having all the answers to client's questions and solutions for all of their problems, things which clients may expect of practitioners. However, enthusiasm for the approach plus knowledge of a few MI strategies is not sufficient to become a proficient practitioner. MI is complex and requires the development of skills over time, similar to any psychological intervention.

Training workshops are offered by accredited trainers around the world (see www.motivationalinterviewing.org). Some are half-day introductory workshops while others are five-day skills-based workshops. Addiction counsellors have usually received extensive training in psychology and/or counselling and will have already developed at least some client-led counselling skills. They are likely to require less training than practitioners in public health settings who are less likely to have acquired counselling skills and may require a shift in their philosophical orientation. The length of training, practice and supervision required to develop the skills required to deliver the MI that fully reflects its spirit may not be practical for many health care professionals (Emmons and Rollnick 2001). It may be more appropriate to train generalist health promoters in BCC. Instruments have been developed to measure proficiency in BCC and MI which can be used for training and research. A behaviour-change counselling index (BECCI) has been developed which can be used for assessing competence in BCC and can be useful for evaluating training (Lane *et al.* 2005). A more extensive instrument, the motivational interviewing skill code (MISC), was developed to study practitioners' proficiency in MI before and after training (Moyes *et al.* 2003). The MISC has been used in a trial of methods to help clinicians improve their proficiency in MI. The study showed that substance abuse professionals can improve their proficiency, both immediately after training and at later follow-up (Miller *et al.* 2004).

Evidence of effectiveness

A number of systematic reviews and meta-analyses have examined the efficacy of MI, the most recent incorporating 72 studies (Rubak *et al.* 2005). Health behaviours covered include drug and alcohol abuse, smoking, diet, exercise, treatment compliance, HIV risk behaviour and the adoption of water purification. Overall, the effect of MI varies widely even within the same health behaviours. This heterogeneity of effects is not explained by study quality, the health behaviour being studied, the quality of MI or session duration, practitioner training or comparison group. The largest effect of MI is reported in studies of drug and alcohol abuse for which it was originally designed. Significant effects are also seen for body mass index, diet and exercise. Perhaps surprisingly, no overall effect has been observed for smoking cessation. The effect of MI seems to increase with additional intervention contacts and interventions that last longer than three months. Its effect also appears to gradually decrease post-intervention. A brief application of MI prior to other treatments or interventions appears to enhance adherence. Consequently, MI might be seen as a complementary intervention to other treatments, rather than as an alternative. Those less ready to change their behaviour tend to respond better to MI than those who are already more ready to change. More traditional behavioural approaches might be more appropriate for the latter group.

So while MI should not be seen as a panacea for all health behaviour interventions, it does produce moderate effects when compared with no treatment or usual care in a range of health behaviours. The variability in effect size limits any conclusions about the particular mechanisms that trigger change. Larger-scale studies with integrated process evaluation may shed light on the most important agents within the MI process. At present the 'active ingredients' of MI remain uncertain and therefore exactly what practitioners need to be trained in and how skilful they need to be remains uncertain. Similarly, limited evidence exists about the effectiveness of MI compared to brief interventions based on other behaviour change theories (see Bandura 2004). Finally, more evidence is required about the effectiveness of MI in minority groups and in a wider variety of cultural settings.

Summary

MI is a style of working with people which emphasizes the quality of the interpersonal relationship and respects a person's autonomy to choose whether or not to change. It does not presume that failure to adopt healthy lifestyles is due to a deficit in knowledge, insight or behavioural skills and, therefore, once these are provided, that behaviour change will follow. Rather, its focus is on the resolution of ambivalence and eliciting intrinsic motivation for change. It is a learnable skill, the proficiency of which can be measured and is appropriate for a range of health behaviours, either as an intervention in its own right or as a complement to other interventions.

References

Bandura A (2004) Health promotion by social cognitive means. *Health Education and Behavior*, 31: 143–64.

Bem DJ (1972) Self-perception theory, in L Berkowitz (ed.) *Advances in Experimental Social Psychology.* New York: Academic Press.

Emmons KM, Rollnick S (2001) Motivational interviewing in healthcare settings: opportunities and limitations. *American Journal of Preventive Medicine,* 20: 68–74.

Harland J, White M, Drinkwater C, Chinn D, Farr L, Howel D (1999) The Newcastle exercise project: a randomised controlled trial of methods to promote physical activity in primary care. *British Medical Journal,* 319: 828–32.

Lane C, Huws-Thomas M, Hood K, Rollnick S, Edwards K, Robling M (2005) Measuring adaptations of motivational interviewing: the development and validation of the behaviour change counselling index (BECCI). *Patient Education and Counseling,* 56: 166–73.

Miller WR, Rollnick S (1991) *Motivational Interviewing: preparing people to change addictive behaviour.* London: Guildford Press.

Miller WR, Rollnick S (2002) *Motivational Interviewing: preparing people for change.* 2nd edition London: Guildford Press.

Miller WR, Yahne CE, Moyers TB, Martinez J, Pirritano M (2004) A randomized trial of methods to help clinicians learn motivational interviewing. *Journal of Consulting and Clinical Psychology,* 72: 1050–62.

Moyes T, Martin T, Catley D, Harris KJ, Ahluwalia JS (2003) Assessing the integrity of motivational interviewing interventions: reliability of the motivational interviewing skills code. *Behavioral and Cognitive Psychotherapy,* 31: 177–84.

Prochaska JO, DiClimente CC, Norcross JC (1992) In search of how people change: applications to addictive behaviours. *American Psychologist,* 47: 1102–14.

Resnicow K, Dilorio C, Soet J, Borrelli B, Hecht J, Ernst D (2002) Motivational interviewing in health promotion: It sounds like something is changing, *Health Psychology,* 21: 444–51.

Rogers CR (1957) The necessary and sufficient conditions for therapeutic personality change. *Journal of Consulting Psychology,* 21: 95–103.

Rubak S, Sandboek A, Lauritzen T, Christensen B (2005) Motivational interviewing: a systematic review and meta-analysis. *British Journal of General Practice,* 55: 305–12.

Tappin DM, Lumsden MA, Gilmour WH, Crawford F, McIntyre D, Stone DH, Webber R, MacIndoe S, Mohammed E (2005) Randomised controlled trial of home based motivational interviewing by midwives to help pregnant smokers quit or cut down. *British Medical Journal,* 331: 373–7.

6 Theatre in health promotion

Overview

In this chapter, you will be introduced to the application of theatre in health promotion and learn how it has evolved since its inception in the 1960s to encompass a wide range of techniques used for different aims and in different settings. You will consider some of the evidence of effectiveness of theatre in health promotion and also learn about best practice in commissioning theatre projects.

Learning objectives

After reading this chapter, you will be better able to:

- **describe the key principles and theory underpinning the use of theatre to promote health**
- **explain when and how to use a range of theatre approaches to promote health**
- **describe the strengths and weaknesses of this method in different settings**
- **commission and evaluate a theatre project in accordance with best practice**

Key terms

Theatre for development Community theatre used both for action research and as a verification tool in development programmes.

Theatre in education (TIE) An umbrella term describing the use of scripted, live theatre usually linked to an interactive workshop used to explore a range of social issues and meet educational aims.

Theatre in health education (THE) Uses the techniques of theatre in education in the service of health education.

Theatre of the oppressed A form of popular theatre of, by and for those engaged in the struggle for liberation. The starting point is not an explicit educational objective, but rather individual and social development and empowerment.

Background and history

'The potential of drama to educate and act as an agent of change has been acknowledged throughout history, but only in the twentieth century has that potential been fully developed' (Wright 1993). The theatre in education (TIE) movement started in the UK in the mid-1960s and developed from the atmosphere of experiment that characterized theatre at that time. Its routes can be traced to the Belgrade Theatre Company, based in the British city of Coventry, which pioneered a participation format for class or small group size as a way of expanding the role of theatre companies and developing relationships with the wider community. The method involved scripted performances plus interactive workshop elements designed to enable participants to engage in critical discussion and analysis of the action.

Changes in education funding led to a decline in TIE projects in the UK during the 1980s. However, since the mid-1990s, TIE has enjoyed a renaissance driven by the rise of new public health approaches and an increasing recognition of the potency of theatre. It is now used as a key method in schools and community settings in attempts to tackle a range of health-related issues. This merging of public health agendas and TIE methodologies led to the term 'theatre in health education' (THE).

However, as funding becomes more closely linked to top-down public health imperatives, TIE and THE practitioners are being given less autonomy to explore issues which may have greater resonance or importance for their target audiences. Some practitioners argue that this has led to a dilution of the quality of projects on offer, and that the *theatre* in TIE and THE is in danger of being relegated by the health education. With the emphasis on personal development, empowerment and problem-solving inherent in THE, there is a possibility that it will fail to recognize drama as an art form with an aesthetic dimension and an impact in itself. Swartzwell (1993) suggests that 'TIE has forgotten that it is theatre'. It is up to health promotion practitioners to ensure that the TIE and THE projects that they commission are developed in a true spirit of partnership with theatre practitioners to ensure a high-quality experience for audiences that will have the most impact, and to avoid drama becoming merely an expensive audio-visual aid.

The wider use of theatre in health promotion

Arts-based methodology are now becoming recognized more widely within public health worldwide, and there has been an emergence of interest in the use of a range of theatre techniques to support public health and development programmes, focusing on traditional 'health' topics and also to support social change.

This is reflected in the range of models of 'theatre in health promotion' that have emerged, and the wider theoretical frameworks used to develop projects: 'Diversification is evident at all levels – ideological, dramaturgical, financial, organisational – it is probably no longer possible to speak of a single TIE movement, but of dialogue between new groupings which needs to be constantly active as new alliances are made' (Jackson 1993).

New types of 'theatre for social change' differ from TIE in the objectives of the work. The purpose of TIE in its traditional form has always been as a method of education, which reflects a philosophical and educational stance. Applied theatre/ theatre for social change uses more than educational theory and seeks to explore, engage with and influence social and cultural norms, and patterns of behaviour. The audience/community participation element is seen as complementary to health promotion strategies and development programmes that aim to empower individuals and communities.

Theatre for development

'The first step to development is a change of attitude, both individual and collective – and in that order – from declared helplessness to empowerment. This is culture in action, and theatre is a cultural tool' (Mavrocordatos 1988). Theatre for development has proved to be an effective way to promote community knowledge and influence behaviour and practice. It is especially useful in remote locations and where there is a tradition of oral communication. It uses and builds upon participatory communication theory, which suggests that projects based on traditional forms of expression have a greater chance of success, as they have cultural resonance and can help to interpret abstract health objectives into a reality for the audiences. When used in development, theatre – as oral communication – creates a 'safe space' in which those who are marginalized can find, and use, a voice to effect change. Performance enables traditionally sensitive and taboo subjects to be voiced, providing a licence to speak which opens doors for future work and so starts the process of development.

Theatre for the oppressed

'Let them create it [solutions to oppression] first in the theatre, in fiction, to be better prepared to create it outside afterwards, for real' (Boal 1979). Augusto Boal created the 'theatre of the oppressed' in the late 1970s. This uses innovative drama techniques to encourage people to address and find solutions to issues of oppression. Boal (2004) defines it as:

> a system of games and special techniques that aims at developing, in oppressed citizens, the language of theatre, which is the essential human language. It is meant to be practised by, about and for the oppressed to help them fight against their oppression and to transform the society that engenders those oppressions. The word oppressed is used in the sense of someone [who] has lost the right to express his or her wills or needs, and is reduced to the conditions of obedient listener of a monologue. It must be used as a tool of fighting against all forms of class oppression, racism, sexism and discrimination. Theatre of the Oppressed does not aim at being only like Hamlet's definition 'a mirror that allows us to see our vices and virtues' but to be an instrument of social transformation.

This type of theatre uses a range of methods and draws upon both active learning theory as well as cognitive behavioural techniques. These include the identification and learning of new ways to behave, cognitive restructuring, and developing new skills to make sense of the world and how we react within it.

Activity 6.1

Read the following brief examples of different types of theatre projects and try to identify what type of 'theatre in health promotion' they represent.

 Example 1: Kolo Village, Mali

The actors have dressed up in the same clothing that the elders wear. One of the actors, a particularly talented mimic, has donned a smock identical to that worn by the chief, and he carries a very similar stick. We see these youths, who have not the license to express their opinions in the ordinary village meetings, begin to address the water crisis. An old man and his family regale the (acted) chief with their tale of woe. Their newly dug well has collapsed. It is March and most of the other wells in the village have run dry. There is much mirth as the husband complains that his food is always late and there is never any water to wash it with – all because his wife spends her entire day queuing for a pot or two of water at the only village pump. [There are] silent smiles at the wife's repartee. (The real chief has a functioning well in his own compound and may not have been so concerned with these problems. A murmur from around as the spectators indicate that they too have realised this.) In response to these supplicants, the (acted) chief summons his elders and they determine to ask the non-governmental organisation (NGO) in the area to donate a tube well. Moving out of the acting area, they make directly for the actual field worker in question who was sitting in the audience. They proceed, effectively, to hold the meeting that they believed the elders should have held – and with complete artistic license. The field worker responds, suggesting that they consider rebuilding some of the wells that are closer to the river. He takes care to point out that if they make the first move, the NGO will respond in their own turn with some technical and material support. The chief takes the message back to his elders.

(Mavrocordatos 1988)

 Example 2: The Lilac Tent, Bolivia

The Lilac Tent experience in Bolivia is inspired by various performing arts and housed under a huge circus travelling tent. The project aims to influence the sexual behaviour of Bolivian youth and prevent the transmission of HIV/AIDS. It is a mixture of entertainment and educational activities and is something like a medieval circus combined with modern educational techniques. Outside the tent people can watch video documentaries on health issues, puppet performances or theatre shows, while inside in groups of 10, visitors have the opportunity of participating in a series of instructive games and activities.

(Dagron 2001)

 Example 3: Crossroads Theatre for Youth (CTY), American Samoa

The goal of CTY is to educate and create awareness of youth and social issues. It uses the process of theatre to inspire imagination, exercise critical thinking, and provoke thought to create solutions to social issues that arise in the local community. The issues based plays are followed by interactive discussion that allow the audience to look at the issues from different perspectives and challenges young people to explore all possible answers and solutions. 'Silent Cries' is a play that runs for 25 minutes and depicts the gradual decline of inter-personal relationships within a family, eroded by substance abuse, family violence, suicide and a total breakdown of any hope in seeing or hearing the reality of what the victims are

experiencing. The performance is followed by a workshop and raises a number of issues that are likely to stay with the audience once the curtain comes down.

(Seui Li'a 2005)

 Example 4: Punjab Lok Rahs

Rahs is a theatre group that cherishes a society that has gender equity and democratic values, respects all human rights and offers equal economic opportunities for all. Rahs believes in organisational and conscious effort to realise this dream. Theatre is its working medium. It has a 15-year history and has written 30 plays, and produced 350 performances, classical epics, quick response street-skits, improvisations with communities and in villages and urban slums. Issues dealt with include child marriage, a woman's right to marry and staged plays against military dictatorship. It draws from local theatre tradition – Rahs being the Punjab word for local forum theatre. All the theatre actively involves local people in participatory theatre experiences.

(Punjab Lok Rahs 2001)

 Feedback

Example 1: theatre for development. The key issue is participatory activities for development and also the partnership and involvement of local NGOs. This work did actually progress over a number of weeks and resulted in progress towards a communal well, which had not previously been on the agenda of the NGO.

Example 2: theatre in health education. A clear health-related message is the focus of the project.

Example 3: theatre in education. The focus is on exploring social issues of resonance to the community.

Example 4: theatre of the oppressed. There is a focus on using participatory theatre techniques to work with disenfranchised groups on issues related to oppression.

Methods used in TIE

A range of dramatic methods are used in TIE and in other theatre forms used to promote health. The most popular techniques include:

- *Forum theatre*: the action is frozen (by the audience or drama group) and the audience is invited on stage to solve problems and redirect the action. This can be a process that takes place as the drama unfolds or, as in theatre of the oppressed, it can take place during a re-running of the play. Having seen the whole story, the audience is invited to consider whether or not the outcome could have been different, and the play is re-run with the audience able to stop it at any point they feel a crucial 'mistake' is being made.
- *Street theatre/invisible theatre*: issue-based scenes performed in public spaces to stimulate interest and discussion regarding particular issues without the public knowing the scenes have been staged.

- *Monologues*: traditionally monologues refer to one-way communication and do not cater for any response from their audience. Monologue followed by skilled facilitation and exploration of issues raised can be effective in moving towards dialogue. It can be particularly useful in putting across factual information as part of a performance, for example in THE projects.
- *Truth-seating and hot-seating*: members of the audience can question and challenge actors 'in role' to explain and elaborate upon the decisions they made in the drama and the impact this had upon them 'in role'.
- *'Cops in the head'*: internal voices that tell us we can't or that we are not good enough are brought to life, challenged and redirected.
- *Image theatre*: participants sculpt pictures onto their bodies to represent and transform situations and relationships.
- *Rainbow of desire*: relationships are deconstructed so as not only to eliminate what we don't want but to explore and embrace ideas about what it is we do want.

Theatre and health promotion theory and practice

 Activity 6.2

Identify which types of theatre could be used to help address these five action areas identified by the World Health Organization (WHO 1984):

1 Improving access to health and building healthy public policy.
2 The development of an environment conducive to health.
3 The strengthening of social networks and social supports and community action.
4 Promoting positive health behaviour skills and appropriate coping strategies.
5 Increasing knowledge and disseminating information.

 Feedback

Power and control, as well as access to knowledge, are recognized as central issues to health promotion, and a critical task of community empowerment is to enable people to define the agenda for themselves in health terms and seize the political initiative to do so. Despite this social model that emphasizes community-level action and empowerment, it remains a field in many areas that is driven by technical, scientific and expert-driven practice. Theatre is a method for both education and social change that can help to redress this balance. For example, theatre for development projects can enable communities to identify barriers to health and find a voice to communicate them and identify potential solutions; theatre of the oppressed techniques can help 'give voice' to marginalized communities and address institutional barriers to access such as racism, sexism and oppression; theatre in education projects can address issues of social injustice or focus on the development of critical thinking and skills by using techniques such as forum theatre; and theatre in health education projects can focus on specific educational objectives related to health, such as the risks of smoking or sexually transmitted infections.

Characteristics of good practice in implementing theatre projects

Using theatre to promote health is not a 'magic bullet' or 'quick fix' but should be seen as one of many potential components in a successful programme of work. An element of partnership between the commissioning body, audience and theatre practitioners is essential and in order to stay true to the roots of TIE, theatre producers must be allowed to develop their craft and address relevant social and political contexts, and not be constrained by a political or social need to cloud over real and important issues. This is the political element of health promotion work that cannot be ignored. A THE play commissioned to address the dangers of HIV/AIDS, for example, will not work unless it addresses the reality of constraints faced by people attempting to take control over their sexual health, and these are many and varied, and often political. In working with a group of lesbian and gay young people, for example, it may be more appropriate to develop a theatre of the oppressed project to allow them to 'give voice' to the realities they face than a THE project about HIV/AIDS. Equally, as discussed previously, the theatre experience in itself needs to be high quality and relevant to the audience to work. Many evaluations of TIE initiatives have focused on the process of project development and implementation and we can learn a great deal from these studies about the conditions that need to be in place for objectives to be met.

 Activity 6.3

While reading the following checklist of characteristics of good practice, adapted from Sawney *et al.* (2003), consider what barriers and opportunities there may be to developing theatre to promote health in your own setting.

There is a consensus within the literature that theatre projects appear to work best and be most effective when:

- they are an integrated part of a wider programmatic approach to promoting health and consolidate learning acquired through previous work;
- the participants are aware of, and committed to, the considerable planning and organization required and there is close liaison with the theatre company through an identified member of staff with good management skills;
- there is a long lead-in time (up to a year is suggested in several studies) and planning and implementation takes place within the same academic year for school-based projects;
- staff or community workers involved attend a preview performance;
- theatre companies provide a teaching/resource pack which outlines preparatory and follow-up activities for teachers or youth workers, and training for staff in how to use the pack;
- interactive workshops/activities are offered after, or are an integral part of, the performance;
- the programme is in itself a high-quality experience of theatre with specialists involved in devising, scripting and performing;
- the actors are credible to the audience, use language the audience can relate to, have similar accents and make reference to local places and current issues;
- the programme has clear aims and objectives that have been developed to address specific misconceptions or issues held by, or identified by and with, the audience;
- the programme is evaluated.

Feedback

If you cannot address the above issues, you should consider alternative options. It may be useful to focus your thoughts by considering:

- Who else needs to be involved?
- Are the building blocks in place to develop theatre projects or are there more immediate priorities before you can develop theatre as part of a programmatic approach?
- What specific aims are you trying to address?
- Why should you use theatre?
- What are the barriers (these might include financial, time, personnel or skills constraints)?
- In addressing barriers, you may then need to consider what training opportunities might exist to develop necessary skills, what funding streams may be available and what local structures are already in place that could support the work (e.g. NGOs, government, educational).
- If it seems unattainable to develop a theatre project at this point, think about what foundations could be laid to enable theatre projects in the future.

Evaluating theatre projects

One of the most problematic areas in the use of theatre to meet health promotion and education aims, and arguably one of the most underdeveloped, is evaluation. Without an evaluation it is not really possible to be sure that you have achieved what you set out to achieve, to be able to demonstrate the value of the work to funders and participants alike, or to learn from the experience to develop practice in the future. Evaluation also enables theatre companies and commissioners of projects to identify any unexpected outcomes that may result from the work.

As you will learn in Chapter 16, evaluation is a multi-faceted process and how it is tackled will depend on what is being evaluated and why, and who is undertaking it and for whom. The following are key elements of good evaluation in theatre projects:

- *Process evaluation*: an ongoing evaluation of the delivery process carried out throughout the life of a project that makes it possible to make assessments along the way about how things are going and therefore make appropriate changes to the work.
- *Impact evaluation*: identifies the immediate achievements of an intervention particularly in relation to the objectives of a piece of work. Objectives should include both instructional objectives (which specify skills and information to be learnt) and expressive objectives, which identify a situation in which a group is to work or a task in which they are to engage, but which do not specify what they are to learn. In the case of TIE projects this provides an opportunity to have objectives related to exploration of issues rather then predetermined learning.
- *Outcome evaluation*: concentrates on identifying the longer-term outcomes.

The complexity of theatre means that its success should not be judged purely on outcomes relating to knowledge, attitudes and behaviour, but also on its ability to create effective dialogue about sensitive issues and to engage appropriately with young people/target audiences (Douglas *et al.* 2000).

 Activity 6.4

Read the following case study of a TIE project and consider how you might evaluate it.

 SEX FM Forum Theatre London

Sex FM is an interactive performance designed to build confidence and teach life skills to young people. It places pupils aged 15 at the heart of the action and encourages them to take part in active discussion about teenage pregnancy and sexually transmitted infections. The performance uses two short stories revolving around the sexual pressures faced by young people. The stories are enacted once in their entirety and then replayed as forum theatre with young people stepping in to stop the action at key points, suggesting different outcomes or decisions to be made by the actors. Each year, teachers and school nurses are invited to in-school teacher training sessions to prepare them for the play. A teaching pack with pre- and post-performance sessions is provided (adapted from Sawney *et al.* 2003).

 Feedback

Questions you might think about in designing your evaluation would include:

*   What are you trying to find out by evaluating the project and how will you use the answers to these questions?
*   What information will give you the answers to your evaluation questions?
*   What tools will you use to collect the information?
*   Who do you want to collect the information from?
*   Who will do the evaluation?

How effective is theatre in health promotion?

While considerable work still needs to be done in developing rigorous evaluations of theatre, a number of studies have explored its effectiveness as a method for addressing personal, social and health-related issues. These studies include peer-reviewed academic research papers and unpublished internal evaluation reports. Some key themes can be drawn from reviews of effectiveness (Sawney *et al.* 2003):

*   *An innovative learning tool*: there is overwhelming agreement that people find theatre to be an engaging, interesting and enjoyable medium for learning and an effective medium for generating discussion about sensitive issues.
*   *Increasing knowledge*: evidence regarding the impact of TIE on the knowledge levels is equivocal. Some studies have observed an increase in knowledge, although improvement was often only slight. Other studies conclude that traditional TIE does not impact on knowledge levels. There is a suggestion that where knowledge levels have improved it is because specific misconceptions have been identified among the audience (Sawney *et al.* 2003). However,

acquisition of knowledge is often not the primary aim of theatre in health promotion. Indeed, lack of evidence of learning may reinforce the need to consider carefully the most appropriate type of theatre to develop in any given setting.

- *Influencing attitudes*: there is some evidence that theatre can be effective in influencing attitudes in a positive way. There is no agreement regarding the degree to which this can happen but several studies suggest that the process of involvement in a dramatic experience is more powerful in influencing emotions and feelings than factual learning.
- *Influencing behaviour*: there is little evidence available on the long-term impact of theatre projects on behaviour. There is, however, a small amount of research that suggests improvements in *intention* and use of strategies explored in theatre to deal with difficult situations after performances.
- *Cost effectiveness*: there have been no cost-effectiveness studies of the use of theatre.

 Activity 6.5

Create a list of potential advantages and disadvantages of the use of theatre considering the particular advantages and disadvantages in your own setting.

 Feedback

The advantages you identified may have included:

- Cultural relevance, especially if led or developed by local troupes or theatre groups.
- Traditional values are preserved and strengthened, and use of local language and idiom contributes to processes of community development and empowerment.
- It allows for the exploration of sensitive or taboo subjects through distancing techniques and scenarios which do not depend on individual disclosure.
- It goes beyond information-giving. Establishing a live dialogue in contrast to other media such as television or radio enables the development of a learning process for the audience, drama groups and project managers.
- Entertainment channels the energy of the audience, through engaging emotions such as surprise, humour and empathy, towards the process of comprehension and participation.
- It engages community/audience.
- It is based on expressed and felt needs.

If done well.

- It is interesting and rewarding.
- Young people in particular are so exposed to the media of television and films that they have built up a degree of immunity to its emotional impact, whereas they often have little or no experience of live drama and its emotional impact.

The disadvantages you identified may have included:

- It is labour intensive in terms of staff and time.
- It is expensive because close rapport and interaction with communities and audiences can only be achieved with small audience sizes so that 'unit costs' are high.

Summary

In this chapter, you have learnt about the various ways in which theatre can be used to support health promotion programmes. There are many different types of theatre and they can complement different elements of a programmatic approach to promoting health. You have learnt about the issues to consider in evaluation as well as what you need to consider in putting theatre projects into practice in your own settings.

References

Boal A (1979) *Theatre of the Oppressed*. London: Pluto Press.
Boal A (2004) International Theatre of the Oppressed website: www.theatreoftheoppressed. org.
Dagron AG (2001) *Making Waves: Stories of Participatory Communication for Social Change*. New York: Rockefeller Foundation.
Douglas N, Warwick I, Whitty G, Aggleton P (2000) Vital youth: evaluating a theatre in health education project. *Health Education*, 100(5): 207–15.
Jackson T (ed.) (1993) *Learning through Theatre*. London: Taylor & Francis.
Mavrocordatos A (1988) Tied up in a rope of sand: theatre for development. Cultural action or development utility paper commissioned for the Contemporary Theatre Review's Issue on Development Theatre in Africa. Winchester: Harwood Academic Publishers (available at www.comminit.com).
Punjab Lok Rahs (2001) www.theatreoftheoppressed.org/uploads//library/evaluations/ info%20PunjabLokRahs.pdf.
Sawney F, Sykes S, Keene M, Swindon L, McCormick G (2003) *It Opened My Eyes – Using Theatre in Education to deliver Sex and Relationships Education*. London: Health Development Agency.
Seui Li'a (2005) Theatre group makes significant strides. *American Alliance for Theatre and Education (AATE) Newsletter*, 5(2). Available from www.aate.org.
Swartzwell L (1993) Trying to like TIE, in T Jackson (ed.) *Learning through Theatre*.
WHO (1984). A discussion document on the concepts and principles of health promotion. Copenhagen: WHO.
Wright P (1993) *An Appraisal of the Uses of Drama in Health Promotion*. Birmingham: The Theatre in Health Education Trust.

Further reading

Kershaw B (1992) *The Politics of Performance: Radical Theatre as a Cultural Intervention*. London: Routledge.
Macdougall J (ed.) (1998) *Contaminating Theatre: Intersections of theatre, therapy and public health*. Evanston, IL: Northwestern University Press.

Useful websites

www.theatreforachange.com
www.tonisant.com – applied and interactive theatre guide
www.artslynx.org
www.art4development.net – arts for global development network
www.ActALIVE.org – email forum for arts for creative transformation
www.theatreoftheoppressed.org – website and email forum containing extensive examples of evaluation reports and literature reviews

7 | Peer education

Overview

This chapter examines what is meant by peer education and outlines some of the theories associated with this approach to health promotion. A number of peer education programmes implemented in different social contexts are then described in order to illustrate the diversity of ways in which peer education can be used. The chapter then draws on evidence from good quality process and outcome evaluations to examine the main issues that should be considered when implementing a peer education programme and the evidence for the effectiveness of the approach.

Learning objectives

After reading this chapter, you will be better able to:

- explain the peer education approach and some of the theories associated with it
- describe some of the key factors that need to be considered in implementing peer education interventions in different social contexts
- discuss findings from both process and rigorous outcome evaluations of peer education interventions and suggest areas for future research

Key terms

Empowerment Individuals are given the knowledge, skills and opportunity to develop a sense of control and mastery over life circumstances.

Peer education The teaching or sharing of information, values and behaviours between individuals with shared characteristics such as behaviour, experience, status or social and cultural backgrounds.

Social learning theory A theory suggesting that individuals learn and then change their behaviour by observing and then modelling the behaviour of others.

Definitions and theories of peer education

Peer education has been defined as the 'teaching or sharing of information, values and behaviours by members of similar age or status group' (Sciacca 1987 cited in Milburn 1995). Researchers and practitioners have drawn on a range of theories to explain the processes involved in peer education, and to justify the use of peer education as a health promotion strategy. The following edited extract from Turner and Shepherd (1999) describes some of the main characteristics of the key theories.

Activity 7.1

When reading this extract, note the key components of each of the theories. Try to identify which components are common to different theories. Think about how these theories might be relevant to peer education.

The theory most often cited is Social Learning Theory. Based on the work of Bandura and colleagues, Social Learning Theory claims that modeling is an important component of the learning process . . . subjects observe behaviour taking place and then go on to adopt similar behaviour. Subjects need an opportunity to practice modeled behaviour and positive reinforcement of it is to be adopted successfully. The extent to which individuals are influenced by modeled behaviour depends on the characteristics of the models, the attributes of the observers and the perceived consequences of adopting similar behaviour . . . Important elements on the learning process are role model credibility and reinforcement of learned behaviour.

Role Theory is based on the concept of social roles and role expectations the idea is that peer educators will adapt to the role expectations of a tutor and behave appropriately. In addition, through adopting a role, individuals develop a deeper understanding and commitment to it. Peer educators can therefore develop a commitment to peer education and the relevance of the health topic. Role theory is based on the premise that communication is inhibited by differences in culture between the teacher and the learner. Peer educators who have a similar set of experiences and culture are therefore likely to be more effective in promoting learning.

Communications of Innovations Theory [or Diffusions of Innovations Theory] explains how innovations come to be adopted by communities and what factors influence the rate of adoption. Such factors include the characteristics of those who adopt the innovation and the characteristics of 'change agents' . . . [it is argued] that all innovations follow a similar pattern of adoption with one group of people – the 'innovators' taking it up immediately . . . then there are the 'early adopters' . . . and finally the laggards, including some who never adopt the innovation. In this theory the 'change agents' influence key 'opinion leaders' within the community. [it is argued] that effective communication occurs when source and receiver are 'homophilous' i.e. are similar in certain attributes such as beliefs, values, education and social status.

Feedback

Common to all these theories is the idea that behaviour is influenced by an individual's social networks and the values and beliefs of peers. The idea is that peers, particularly those who are considered 'role models' or 'opinion leaders', are able to communicate information in credible and appealing ways. Shared social norms means that peers can present information, and even model values and behaviours, with greater social and cultural relevance so that this is likely to influence the health-related behaviours of others.

As well as theories that inform and explain peer education, some authors have attempted to develop systems of classifying peer education interventions according to specific dimensions. For example, Wilton *et al.* (1995) describe a categorization which suggests that peer-delivered health promotion interventions can differ according to the extent to which they are initiated and driven by health professionals (top-down) or peer groups themselves (bottom-up), and the extent to which they employ informal (unstructured with peer educators taking an active role) or formal methods (content is prescribed by others and approach is didactic). Others have described peer approaches in terms of the extent to which they incorporate formal pedagogical approaches; use diffusional techniques so that education occurs as part of the usual peer interaction that occurs in social groups; and/or involve community mobilization where people become active members of their community and in doing so educate others (Svenson 1998).

Examples of peer education in different contexts

Interventions involving peer education are diverse and have been implemented with different groups of people (e.g. young people, men who have sex with men, commercial sex workers), in various social contexts (e.g. schools, prisons, workplaces and villages), in developed and developing countries, and addressing a range of health topics (e.g. HIV prevention, smoking and drug use prevention, asthma management and mental health). Three peer education projects are described below in order to illustrate the diversity of interventions involved.

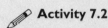 **Activity 7.2**

As you read the following examples of peer education projects, think about how these might be classified according to Wilton *et al.*'s (1995) criteria of using 'bottom-up'/'top-down' approaches and 'informal'/'formal' methods. To what extent might they be considered to: a) incorporate formal pedagogical approaches; b) use diffusional techniques; c) involve community mobilization (Svenson 1998)? How useful are these ways of categorizing approaches to peer education?

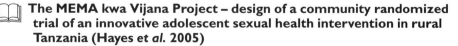 **The MEMA kwa Vijana Project – design of a community randomized trial of an innovative adolescent sexual health intervention in rural Tanzania (Hayes et al. 2005)**

The project is being carried out in 20 rural communities located in four districts of the Mwanza region in north-western Tanzania. The intervention has four components, the main one being a teacher-led, peer-assisted programme of lessons on sexual health delivered in the last three years of primary school. Curriculum design is based on the principles of social learning theory and aims to provide basic knowledge, improve perceptions of risk, encourage adoption of safer sexual behaviour, provide sexual negotiation skills and challenge commonly held gender stereotypes, such as the belief that girls cannot refuse sex if they have received a gift. Lessons are highly participatory and involve the use of drama, stories, role-plays, games and internalization exercises. Teachers are trained to deliver the programme and are assisted by trained peer educators elected by their classmates, whose main functions are to perform a series of short dramas, acting as discussion starters and to assist with role-plays.

 ### HIV/AIDS prevention among the male population: results of a peer education program for taxicab and tricycle drivers in the Philippines (Morisky et al. 2005)

The intervention sites were Lapu-Lapu and Mandawe City, two large cities in the southern Philippines. Both taxi and tricycle drivers' associations operating in these cities participated in the study. The owners and officers of the taxicab and tricycle associations were informed of the nature of the proposed intervention programme. Seminars were carried out with taxicab and tricycle drivers. These covered STI/HIV/AIDS, sexuality, methods of transmission and prevention (with an emphasis on condom use) and the role of men in transmission. Slides and video presentations, as well as guided model demonstrations and self reinforcements, were used to equip individuals with basic knowledge and skills. Prior to the conclusion of the seminar, 20 peer educators from each target group were recruited by group nomination, volunteer and/or appointed by their officials. These peer educators underwent an additional two days' training. They were taught methods to engender communications skills so that they could influence other drivers to educate their customers on the importance of safer sexual practices as well as provide condoms to their customers. The peer educators then developed educational materials (e.g. posters and stickers) and taught their peers at different sites such as the tricycle drivers at the terminals while waiting for passengers. The intention was that as well as changing the knowledge and behaviour of taxi and tricycle drivers who tend to visit commercial sex workers, they will influence the knowledge and behaviour of their clients who request entertainment information from them. The peer educators continued to meet monthly with the site coordinator to discuss problems encountered, successful approaches and share strategies.

 ### Pupil-led sex education in England (RIPPLE study): cluster randomized intervention trial (Stephenson et al. 2004)

The intervention was designed by an external team of health promotion practitioners with experience of delivering peer led sexual health programmes in UK schools . . . The programme was piloted to ensure that it was acceptable to teachers and pupils and could be implemented in a fairly standardised way across different types of schools. The programme was not designed explicitly around any particular theoretical framework. Volunteer peers educators were recruited from Year 12 (aged 16/17 years). The peer educators carried out a needs assessment exercise with Year 9 pupils and were then trained to prepare classroom sessions aimed at improving the younger pupils' skills in sexual communication and condom use, and their knowledge about pregnancy, STI, contraception and local sexual health services. The peer educators were also supported to prepare lesson plans and identify resources. Ongoing support was provided by teachers who organised suitable times for teams of peer educators to deliver three sessions of SRE to Year 9 pupils. Teachers were not present in the classroom. Each session lasted around one hour, and used participatory learning methods and activities focusing on relationships, STI and contraception.

Feedback

Often evaluation reports of peer education interventions provide limited information about the approach used by peer educators and/or the content of the intervention. While useful as a framework, one limitation of the classification system suggested by Wilton *et al.* is that the 'formal/informal' definition appears to encapsulate two dimensions. For example, the content of a peer education intervention may be mostly prescribed by those other than the peer educators (considered 'formal') but the approach for delivering this information may not necessarily be didactic. Interventions may not easily be defined as 'top-down' or 'bottom-up'; methods used for delivering information (e.g. by contacting drivers at the terminals while waiting for passengers or using peers in classroom sessions) may be decided by intervention organizers but the content of the interventions may be decided by the educators themselves.

Many interventions may incorporate elements of all the different approaches proposed by Svenson (1998). When assessing the extent to which an intervention may be considered to include 'formal pedagogical approaches', it is necessary to consider the usual pedagogical approaches used in the particular social context. For example, in some schools, and in some countries, teacher-led lessons may be highly participatory (and perhaps involve the use of drama and role play) while in other schools this may be very unusual. The meaning, acceptability and impact of participatory approaches is likely to be different in these different contexts. Deciding whether an intervention involved diffusional techniques may depend on how the boundaries of the intervention are defined. For example, students who have participated in a classroom session led by peer educators may then share this information with their peers during their normal social interaction.

Evidence from process evaluations

Process evaluations aim to examine how interventions are delivered and received and why an intervention might or might not be effective (see Chapter 15). The findings of process evaluations provide important information about the factors most likely to determine the success of peer-delivered approaches in different contexts. The following draws on evidence from process evaluations and findings from the systematic review by Harden *et al.* (1999), to examine the main issues that should be considered when designing and implementing a peer education programme.

Needs assessments

As you have learnt, identifying the needs of the target group is an important component in the development of health promotion interventions and broadly 'needs' can be considered in terms of those a group itself says and feels should be addressed, or those which 'experts' identify as being important. Engaging a population in assessing its own needs and formulating responses to these is particularly important in the development of interventions, such as peer education, that adopt an empowerment-based approach. However, Harden *et al.* (1999) found that assessment of reported needs is not a common feature of peer-delivered interventions with young people. Only 4 of 49 outcome evaluations and 2 out of 15 process evaluations that were reviewed incorporated an assessment of the reported needs of the target group. Well over half of the evaluations explicitly stated that the intervention was based on normative needs.

Formative research

As well as assessments of health promotion needs, it is important to assess participants' preferences for methods of provision as well as the desired topics to be addressed by the intervention. This is often a neglected part of intervention development. For example, although peer educators in the RIPPLE study carried out a needs assessment with the target group focusing on the topics that pupils might like to have covered in the lessons, no research or consultation was undertaken regarding how the intervention was to be delivered. The process evaluation later found that although all peer education was delivered in mixed-sex classes, most girls and a third of boys would have preferred at least some of the classes to be delivered in single-sex groups (Strange *et al.* 2003).

Formative research can also be important in assessing how a particular intervention, found effective in one context, might need to be amended to be successfully implemented in another. One example of this is a peer-delivered intervention where 'popular opinion leaders' were recruited to serve as HIV prevention peer educators in gay bars in various US cities (Kelly *et al.* 1997). When transferred to bars in Glasgow in Scotland and gyms in London, similar interventions were found to be ineffective. Process evaluation suggested these new interventions were hindered, respectively, by bars being inappropriate settings in which to discuss personal sexual behaviour, and peer educators in gyms finding it difficult to approach men, most of whom were complete strangers to them (Hart and Elford 2003).

Engaging stakeholders

It is important to engage all relevant stakeholders when planning and implementing a peer education project, particularly where these involve setting laws and policies and providing access to services. Stakeholders may also be influential in ensuring continued funding and the ongoing sustainability of programmes. Enabling peer educators to make decisions about the direction and content of interventions may require sensitive negotiation with stakeholders who may wish to influence the aims and objectives of an intervention and who may find giving up control of resources (and power) difficult.

Recruiting peer educators

The way in which individuals are recruited as peer educators is important as it determines the types of people who become peer educators and the commitment they have to a project. Decisions about who to recruit are complicated by a lack of clarity about what makes someone a 'peer'. Furthermore, the different theoretical perspectives outlined above may result in different approaches to recruitment. For example, theories emphasizing diffusional processes may suggest that those who are most similar to the target group in terms of status or values are recruited, while theories focusing on processes of community mobilization might suggest that recruiting 'opinion leaders' may be more effective.

Approaches to recruiting peer educators have included: providing information about a project and then asking for volunteers, for example in school assemblies (Stephenson *et al.* 2004); identifying and approaching popular 'opinion leaders' from among target groups; and asking members of the target groups to nominate peers. A further technique, which acknowledges the complexity of social networks and the existence of cultural sub-groups, is to ask a target group to identify the various sub-groups and then to select peer educators from each of these on the basis of self-defined membership of such sub-groups.

Harden *et al.* (1999) found that in projects working with young people, most used some kind of selection criteria for recruiting peer educators and that this commonly resulted in peer educators that were high academic achievers. Peer educators in the RIPPLE study were recruited from Year 12 (aged 16/17 years). Although they were volunteers and were not selected using any specific criteria, they were older than the young people to whom they delivered the sex education classes. They were also higher academic achievers and were more likely to be white, female and from less socioeconomically disadvantaged backgrounds. The possibility that these individuals were not really 'peers' of many of the younger students constituting the target groups was suggested as a contributing factor to the limited success of the intervention. Most studies reviewed by Harden *et al.* reported that recruiting male peer educators is more difficult than recruiting females. A few studies have specifically recruited peer educators from 'hard-to-reach' groups, though this is unusual and requires project workers to make specific efforts to contact and engage these groups of people. Fox *et al.* (1993) aimed to provide young people in schools with insight into issues connected with early parenthood. Peer educators were young mothers who youth workers contacted outside of the school setting. These mothers then collaborated with the youth workers to set the aims and develop the content of the intervention.

Harden *et al.* report that it is not clear from the existing evidence who or what types of people make the best peer educators. Studies have reported that peer educators have most impact on those who resemble them in terms of age, sex, ethnicity and school status. However, there is also evidence to suggest that peer educators' experience of the topic in question, the way that they deliver their message and their personality may actually be more important than their demographic characteristics. It is possible that the relative importance of demographic similarity, experience of the topic and personality type might be dependent on the specific setting that the peer education is occurring in, the groups of people involved and the health issue being addressed.

Training peer educators

Many studies emphasize the importance of adequate training for peer educators, although there is no clear evidence about the optimum amount of training that is required in different contexts. Generally, peer educators report satisfaction with training, although Harden *et al.* found that young people acting as peer educators sometimes report not feeling adequately prepared to work with groups of their peers, particularly in school settings. Providing skills in classroom and/or group management may be particularly important in determining the success of these types of peer education interventions, as studies report peer leaders as being better received by their target groups when they are thought to be well prepared and confident with class control. Designing the training required to equip people to deliver health promotion messages first requires decisions to be made concerning, for example, how formal or informal the methods to be used by the peer educators should be. Harden *et al.* suggest that while peer educators are often trained using approaches common to counselling, the methods that they are taught to use with those they are educating are often more formal and in line with standard teaching methods. This has implications for the way in which they are likely to interact and communicate with their peers and therefore for the likely success of the intervention. The use of counselling techniques when training peer educators may also partly explain why peer educators report such enhanced feelings of empowerment and self-efficacy (Harden *et al.* 1999). Regardless of the formality of the approach taken, ongoing support and training is important in order to help peer educators consolidate their skills, share strategies that have been found to be successful and get advice on issues that arise as projects unfold (Morisky *et al.* 2005).

Utilizing informal and existing interactions between people

Peer education's use of existing modes of communication and equitable power relations between people are regarded as two of its main strengths (Turner and Shepherd 1999). However, the reality of both these features of peer-delivered interventions have been challenged. In relation to sexual health interventions with young people, Walker (1994) found that young people often felt constrained by gendered expectations in terms of how they felt able to talk about sex and sexuality with peers. Frankham (1998) has questioned the extent to which young people do actually talk about sex in ways that would facilitate the communication of health information in informal contexts. While such difficulties with communicating health information may be particular to socially sensitive topics, such as sexual health, they are not only found among young people. Flowers and Hart (1999) report that gay men recruited as peer educators found it difficult to broach discussion of personal sexual behaviour and sexual health needs with men in bars. Research suggests that how young people interact in the course of peer education in schools is determined by the context and prevailing culture within the school. For example, young people often become 'teacherly' in their relations with peers because teachers are the only available, situated model for educating others (Frankham 1998). These examples highlight the importance of considering the social context in which peer education is likely to be carried out and the impact of this on the type of communication that can occur.

Power and relations between health professionals and target groups

One of the main justifications for engaging peer educators in health promotion is that this can empower target groups by enabling people to participate in actively defining and addressing their own health needs. The idea of empowerment and participation enhancing the impact of an intervention is in line with some of the fundamental principles of health promotion. However, genuine empowerment requires health professionals to work in equitable partnership with target groups, thereby relinquishing some of their own power.

Projects where heath professionals have worked in partnership with target groups have been successfully implemented. For example, Kegeles *et al.* (1996) report on a community-based HIV prevention intervention with young gay men where a core group of such men sat on a decision-making body designing the content of materials and the methods used for intervention delivery. However, evidence suggests that most peer education projects do not incorporate a genuinely equitable relationship between health professionals and their target groups.

Tensions can arise between the ideology that peer educators should 'own' and exercise control over the direction of projects and professionals' views about what are appropriate activities for peer educators to be involved in. Harden *et al.* (1999) report that most projects involving peer educators are top-down rather than bottom-up in that they do not involve members of the target group in the project planning and decision-making and nor do they include any assessment of the needs or interests of the group targeted. With funding for projects controlled by health professionals and usually linked to particular aims and outcomes, and with difference in values between target groups and health professionals often being difficult to reconcile, genuinely bottom-up peer education may be difficult to achieve. It is possible that rather than nurturing empowerment and participation, some peer education may simply involve peers in order that the views, attitudes and values of project organizers can be communicated in ways that are superficially more acceptable to a target population.

Addressing poverty and gender inequalities

Most interventions involving peer education that aim to empower individuals do so through their active participation in programme activities. However, the approach has been criticized for ignoring wider factors that impact on empowerment. Some authors have illustrated how wider social factors, such as hierarchical social relationships in schools, and structural inequalities relating to poverty and gender, can limit the capacity for individuals participating in peer education projects to develop the critical thinking, consciousness-raising and empowerment skills which, it is argued, are required for a programme to be effective. A few peer education projects have directly addressed gendered power relations. The example outlined above (Morisky *et al.* 2005) illustrates a peer-delivered intervention with male taxi and tricycle drivers which recognized the way in which men dominate and control women's sexual behaviour in the Philippines and aimed to address men's social norms in order to influence HIV incidence. Previous interventions with female commercial sex workers concluded that work with their male clients was necessary if women were to be able to practise safer sex.

Satisfaction with peer education

Generally process evaluations find high levels of satisfaction with peer education. For example, students experiencing the RIPPLE intervention described peer educators, compared with teachers, as having: greater relevant expertise; more respect for students; being more confident, empathetic and trustworthy; holding more similar values about sex; using familiar 'slang' language; being less moralistic; and being better at making the sessions fun. Harden *et al.* (1999) reported that very few of the process evaluations reviewed included any negative comments or criticism from participants. However, the findings of these studies may be subject to information bias and it is difficult to draw conclusions about how representative the views gathered from small numbers of interviews and focus groups are of the wider population. The RIPPLE study found that, in focus groups, students were very positive about peer sex education. However, data collected in questionnaires indicated that a third did not evaluate the sex education positively. Various schools-based evaluations (including the RIPPLE study) have highlighted students concerns about peer educators being unable to manage disruptive students.

As peer educators often use participative methods and peer education programmes may address different issues than conventional non-peer delivered programmes, it is difficult to identify whether participants' satisfaction is a consequence of involving peer educators or of the different methods employed and issues addressed. In the RIPPLE study the teaching methods used by the peer educators often involved a lot of classroom activity and small group work, which students said made it easier for them to participate and verbally contribute to the sessions. The content of the sessions was seen as more relevant than lessons they had had with teachers. Students felt they were learning something new, in a new format.

The acceptability of many of the methods used by peer educators in projects in high-income countries to participants in projects being implemented in low-income countries has still to be established. The use of interactive and participative teaching strategies, such as modelling of behaviour through role play or changing social norms through use of drama, may not be acceptable in some cultures. These approaches may be particularly inappropriate where people are unfamiliar with such teaching strategies and where public discussion of sexual matters can result in individuals being stigmatized. The possibility that these methods may not be appropriate highlights the potential difficulty of transferring approaches based on theories (such as social learning theory) that have been developed in the developing world to very different social contexts.

Costs and sustainability

Developing ways of achieving long-term financial sustainability for peer education projects has been identified as an issue of concern for those involved in organizing and implementing programmes. There are various ways in which financial sustainability can be achieved by programmes, for example through methods of income generation such as clinic fees or condom sales. Some programmes have attempted to increase their sustainability by integrating peer education into schools' existing curricula. In addition, there is potential for community funds to be created, for example from the interest on small loans provided as part of micro-credit schemes such as village banking programmes.

Much of the literature highlights the importance of incentives for peer educators. Incentives are considered important to encourage people to volunteer and also to ensure their continuing involvement and therefore the ongoing sustainability of a project. While peer educators may wish for some compensation for their time and involvement in projects, programme organizers should consider the possible impact of providing incentives on their status as peers. The provision of quite basic resources such as T-shirts or free meals may undermine the status of individuals as it may differentiate them from the individuals whom they are educating.

 Activity 7.3

Imagine you have been asked to design a peer education programme to increase levels of exercise by young people (aged 11–16 years). How might you go about designing such an intervention? What are the key issues you would need to resolve?

 Feedback

Key questions to consider when designing such an intervention might include:

- Who are the 'target group' of young people (e.g. age, sex, socioeconomic status, living in which areas)?
- Who are considered their 'peers'?
- How much and what types of exercise do these young people engage in currently and what types of exercise are they interested in?
- What services currently exist and what are the barriers for young people in accessing these?
- What existing literature can provide insights into these issues and what additional information should be collected?
- What is the budget for the proposed intervention and which stakeholders (e.g. funders, providers of sports services, teachers, parents, young people) should be involved in the planning of the intervention?
- How involved in the planning, implementation and decision-making should the target young people and their peers be and how will this be achieved?
- Which aims and objectives of the intervention are prescribed?
- What type of interaction between peers and the target group of young people is being aimed for and what are the implications for recruiting, training and supporting peer educators?
- What aspects of the proposed intervention should be piloted?
- How can the feasibility, accessibility, acceptability and impact of the intervention be evaluated?
- What measures could be put in place to ensure the (financial) sustainability of the programme?

Evidence from outcome evaluations

Impacts on target groups

Conclusions regarding the potential effectiveness of peer-delivered approaches are best made on the basis of systematic reviews of rigorously designed studies such as randomized controlled trials (RCTs) or matched comparison studies. To date, the systematic review of peer-delivered health promotion with young people by Harden *et al.* (1999) is the only published review available that focuses solely on peer education interventions. It found just 12 studies designed in such a way that reliable conclusions about effectiveness could be drawn. Few well conducted randomized trials were undertaken, and none were implemented in developing countries. Of those studies that were included in the review, more than half found a positive effect of peer education on at least one behavioural outcome. The effective interventions, and the contexts in which these were carried out, were diverse. For example, effective interventions included those delivered in community and school settings and those that focused on topics such as sexual health, smoking and violence. Some effective interventions employed a community mobilization approach and others involved a more formal pedagogical approach.

Effective interventions also differed in the methods used for recruiting peer educators and the amount of training provided to them. This diversity in the approaches employed by and the characteristics of effective peer education programmes may illustrate the importance of interventions responding to the specific characteristics of the social context in which they are implemented and the needs of the target groups involved in order to be effective. None of the sexual health interventions included in the systematic review were implemented in school settings. The findings of phase one of the RIPPLE study (students were aged 16 years) found that in comparison to teacher-led sex education, peer education increased young people's knowledge, increased girls' confidence in using condoms and their confidence in saying no to unwanted sexual activity. The intervention had no effect on condom or contraception use, regret at first sex, or quality of first sexual experience or relationship. Girls were however less likely to report having had heterosexual sex.

As well as establishing which characteristics of peer education programmes might be most important in determining effectiveness, it is also useful to know for which sub-groups of target populations an intervention may be most effective. Harden *et al.* (1999) found that the effects of interventions were often limited to particular sub-groups, often those who were least at risk of poor health outcomes. An example cited found that a school-based smoking prevention intervention was only effective for females who were non-smokers at age 11. Evidence from outcome evaluations that also included process evaluations suggests that this may be because interventions are less acceptable to those most at risk and who may also be less likely to participate or engage with an intervention (Kegeles *et al.* 1996). Findings from sub-group analyses should be interpreted with care as repeated post hoc statistical testing increases the likelihood of finding significant results by chance.

Impact on peer educators

Many studies report a positive impact on peer educators' knowledge, skills and personal development. This is sometimes presented as a major justification for the implementation of peer education programmes. Only a few studies report no positive effects resulting from involvement as a peer educator. However, no studies have evaluated the impact of peer education programmes on outcomes for peer educators using an appropriately rigorous study design, such as the RCT, that would enable firm conclusions about effectiveness to be drawn. Further research examining effects of participation on peer educators using appropriate research designs would be useful.

 Activity 7.4

Design an RCT with an integral process evaluation to assess the feasibility, acceptability, accessibility and effectiveness of the peer education programme for taxi and tricycle drivers in the Philippines (see p. 100). What might be the key challenges when implementing this evaluation?

 Feedback

A number of 'similar' cities could be identified, recruited to the study and randomized to either a comparison or intervention group. Adequate numbers of cities and men should be recruited to the study for the desired change in outcome (HIV status or more likely a proxy indicator for this) to be identified (this can be done by performing a 'power calculation'). A process evaluation could use methods such as questionnaires and interviews to gather the perspectives of all the key stakeholders including owners of the taxicab and tricycle associations, drivers, peer educators and their clients (male passengers). Data about the feasibility, accessibility and acceptability of the intervention should be collected. Data about any existing HIV/AIDS prevention interventions that might impact on the target group in the comparison cities should also be collected. Baseline (pre-intervention) and outcome data should be collected from a random sample of the target group in both intervention and comparison cities post-intervention and at appropriate follow-ups (e.g. each year etc.). Challenges when designing and implementing this evaluation might include: identifying and recruiting adequate numbers of 'similar' cities; developing appropriate methods for ensuring that participants in the study can provide informed consent for participation in the intervention and/or research activities; deciding what information about the aims and design of the study should be presented to research participants; deciding the extent to which the peer-led intervention should be standardized across cities; choosing appropriate methods for monitoring the peer education intervention in comparison cities; and ensuring that individuals from whom baseline data are collected can be re-contacted to assess outcomes.

Summary

Peer education interventions have become immensely popular with practitioners and have incorporated a diverse range of approaches and addressed a wide variety of health issues. A range of, mostly psychosocial, theories have been drawn on to justify the use of peer education as a health promotion strategy and to explain some of the processes involved. Process evaluations suggest that future interventions might be improved through the incorporation of needs assessments that enable the target population to assess their own expressed needs, and formative evaluation that assesses the feasibility and acceptability of the intervention to all members of the target group, particularly those at most risk of adverse health outcomes. Those implementing peer education projects should be aware that the method of recruitment will impact on the type of people who ultimately become peer educators. Involving those from 'hard-to-reach' groups as peer educators will require particular effort and resources. Process evaluations have also highlighted the challenges for health professionals of working with target groups in ways that involve them in decision-making processes, nurture their ownership of interventions and genuinely facilitate their empowerment. Whether or not peer education projects really can 'empower' individuals may depend on their ability to address wider structural inequalities, such as those related to gender and poverty.

Finally, this chapter has also highlighted the need for more well-designed and rigorously implemented evaluations (e.g. using RCT designs) to assess the effectiveness of peer education interventions, particularly in developing countries.

References

Flowers P, Hart G (1999) Everyone on the scene is so cliquey: are gay bars an appropriate context for a community-based peer-ed intervention? in P Aggleton, G Hart, P Davies (eds) *Families and Communities Responding to AIDS*. London: UCL Press.

Fox J, Walker B, Kushner S (1993) *'It's not a bed of roses': young mothers' education project evaluation report*. Norwich: Centre for Applied Research in Education, University of East Anglia.

Frankham J (1998) Peer education: the unauthorized version. *British Educational Research Journal*, 24: 179–93.

Harden et al. (1999) *A Review of the Effectiveness and Appropriateness of Peer-delivered Health Promotion Interventions for Young People*. London: EPI Centre Social Science Research Unit.

Hart G, Elford J (2003) The limits of generalisability: community-based sexual health interventions among gay men, in J Stephenson et al. (eds) *Effective Sexual Health Interventions: issues in experimental evaluation*. Oxford: Oxford University Press.

Hayes RJ et al. (2005) The MEMA kwa Vijana Project: design of a community randomized controlled trial of an innovative adolescent sexual health intervention in rural Tanzania. *Contemporary Clinical Trials*, 26(4): 430–42.

Kegeles SM, Hays RB, Coates TJ (1996) The empowerment project: a community level HIV prevention intervention for young gay men. *American Journal of Public Health*, 86(8): 1129–36.

Kelly JA, Murphy DA, Sikkema KJ, McAuliffe TL, Roffman RA, Solomon LJ, Winett RA, Kalichman SC (1997) Randomized controlled community level HIV prevention and intervention for sexual risk behavior among homosexual men in US cities. *Lancet*, 350: 1500–5.

Milburn K (1995) A critical review of peer education with young people with special reference to sexual health. *Health Education Research*, 10(4): 407–20.

Morisky *et al.* (2005) HIV/AIDS prevention among the male population: results of a peer education program for taxicab and tricycle drivers in the Philippines. *Health Education and Behaviour*, 32(1): 57–68.

Stephenson JM, Strange V, Forrest S, Oakley A, Copas A, Allen E, Babiker A, Black S, Ali M, Johnson AM and the RIPPLE Study team (2004) Pupil-led sex education in England (RIPPLE study): cluster randomized intervention trial. *Lancet*, 364: 338–46.

Strange V, Forrest S, Oakley A and the RIPPLE study team (2003) Mixed or single sex education: how would people like their sex education and why? *Gender and Education*, 15: 201–14.

Svenson GR (1998) *Annotated Bibliography about Youth AIDS Peer Education in Europe*. Sweden: European Commission.

Turner G, Shepherd J (1999) A method in search of a theory: peer education and health promotion. *Health Education Research*, 14(2): 235–47.

Walker B (1994) *No One to Talk With: Norfolk Young People's Conversations about Sex a Basis for Peer Education*. Norwich: Centre for Applied Research in Education, University of East Anglia.

Wilton T, Keeble S, Doyle L, Walsh A (1995) *The Effectiveness of Peer Education in Health Promotion: Theory and Practice*. Bristol: Faculty of Health and Community Studies, University of the West of England.

8 | Mass media campaigns

Overview

In this chapter you will explore the use of mass communication in health promotion. You start by considering the different ways that the mass media influence health, both positively and negatively, and discuss the ways that it has been utilized to advance public health. You go on to look at different models which attempt to explain how the mass media exert their effect. The focus is on the purposive use of mass media channels for health education and health promotion and you will consider the features of effective interventions and the strengths and weakness of the approach. Finally, you will consider some of the issues and debates surrounding the use of the mass media to promote health and some of the challenges that this presents for evaluation.

Learning objectives

After reading this chapter, you will be better able to:

- compare and contrast different models of how the mass media exert their effect
- explain the important elements required in developing mass communication interventions
- describe the strengths and limitations of mass communication in health promotion
- explain the importance of evaluating mass communication and the challenges that evaluation presents

Key terms

Background noise Influences on the target audience other than the intervention, which make it difficult to attribute outcomes to the intervention.

Diffusion acceleration The rapidity with which messages may be disseminated, once the process of transmission from one, to two or more, agencies has begun.

Edutainment Learning through media, particularly mass media, that both educates and entertains.

Mass media Electronic and print channels through which information is transmitted to a large number of people at a time.

Multiplier effect The additional impact achieved when an intervention uses several agencies to pass on a message, each of which convey the message to several other agencies and so on.

Introduction

Mass communication strategies have been used throughout the world in health promotion with varying degrees of success. Interventions on the television, radio and in newspapers have variously sought to promote condom use, hand-washing, breastfeeding and screening services (to name but a few). They have also sought to reduce rates of drug and alcohol misuse, smoking and stigma around diseases such as leprosy and AIDS (again, to name but a few). The last few decades have seen rapid developments in communication technologies, which have resulted in new media channels being opened to health promoters. The internet and mobile phones are being increasingly used as a medium through which health-related messages can be transmitted (e.g. a project in the UK where young women are sent text messages to remind them to take their contraceptive pill). Despite the widespread use of mass communication in health promotion, it remains controversial. It has been argued that such interventions are a waste of money and divert resources away from where they are really needed at the community level, and that many mass communications are about 'selling' health rather than empowering choice and therefore stand on shaky ethical ground (Tones and Green 2004). It is also argued that they tend to be used in the service of individual behaviour change rather than addressing the wider determinants of health, and as a result can be victim-blaming ('we've *told* you what do to; it is *your* fault if you don't do it and so you will have to suffer the consequences', so the argument goes). In this respect they suit politicians, who want to be seen to be doing something.

However, it is universally acknowledged that the mass media are a powerful force for change (both positive and negative) and that the media have a powerful norming function and socialization effect.

 Activity 8.1

Think back over the last two or three days. What have you read, seen or heard that contained messages or information about health issues via the different media identified above?

 Feedback

You may have read a newspaper article on a local rubbish dump polluting the water supply, or seen an advert for cigarettes on a bill-board. Perhaps you heard a radio phone-in on sexual health or watched your favourite soap opera where the main character's drinking is causing trouble at home. Or maybe you saw a government-sponsored poster promoting condom use.

These examples illustrate the many ways that information is generated and transmitted via the mass media. The examples do not all have a direct health-driven agenda, and the impact on health may be an 'incidental byproduct' when the real goal is to sell commercial products or increase viewing figures. In terms of public health, both the 'purposive' and 'incidental' health messages are important. The role of mass media in health can be considered as falling into two categories, as identified by Finnegan and Viswanath (1997).

First, the effects of day-to-day interaction with the media on health outcomes. Research has explored the effects of day-to-day interaction with the mass media on a number of health-related behaviours, for example on violence, eating patterns, tobacco and alcohol use, and more recently on sexual attitudes and behaviours (Escobar-Chaves *et al.* 2005). Studies have tended to focus on two main areas of concern: first, on the nature and extent of media consumption and its influence on attitudes and behaviour; and second on the media portrayal of health issues and their influence on how people see the world (norm-sending). It should be noted here, however, that the effects of day-to-day interaction with the media are not all necessarily negative. We know that the media are an important source of information for many and that messages portrayed may be health-enhancing. Efforts have been, and continue to be, made to engage with programme-makers (both TV and radio) and journalists to influence the way that health issues are portrayed in the media and it is here that the boundaries between the effects of day-to-day interaction and purposive use of the media become blurred.

Second, the effects of the purposive use of the media to achieve some health outcome. At its very simplest the purposive use of the media involves utilizing media channels to transmit messages. Conventionally, this has involved high-profile adverts on the TV, radio or in print media with the aim of changing knowledge, attitudes or behaviour. The repertoire of purposive uses of the mass media has, however, expanded in recent years to include a range of activities from entertainment (learning through media that both educates and entertains, such as soap operas) to media advocacy (the strategic use of mass media for advancing social or public policy goals – see Chapter 9).

It is this purposive use of the media that is the focus of this chapter. But before you learn about this in more detail, you will first touch on the communication process and some of the theories and models of how the mass media may exert its effect.

Communication

Communication is essentially concerned with the transmission and reception of messages. It consists of three components: a sender, a message and a receiver. The sender constructs (or encodes) the message and the receiver makes sense of it (or decodes). Encoded messages can take three forms – symbolic (the spoken or written word), iconic (pictorial) and enactive (communication resulting from the active involvement of the receiver). The process of decoding also involves three stages. First, the message must reach the receiver; second, the receiver must pay attention to it; and third, the message must be correctly interpreted. When the message is transmitted via the mass media it is mediated and the sender is not present, so there is the potential for the message to be understood in a way other than intended. This is one of the reasons why formative research is so important in mass communications (see evaluation below).

 Activity 8.2

Using one of the examples you identified in Activity 8.1, try to identify who was the sender of the message. How did they 'encode' the message and what did you understand the message to be? On reflection, could the message have been interpreted in a different way?

 Feedback

How a message is perceived and interpreted will depend on a number of factors, including who the source of the message is believed to be and whether they are seen as credible or not.

How does the mass media exert its effect?

Glover (1984 cited in Naido and Wills 1994) proposes four models for how the media exert their effect:

- *Direct effects or 'hypodermic syringe'*: this model assumes the existence of a passive audience on whom the mass media can have a direct effect. Messages are 'injected' into the population. This model has been widely rejected. In the 1960s, for example, Mendelsohn saw mass media approaches more in terms of a diffuse aerosol spray with a 'hit and miss' effect: 'we now begin to look at mass communications as a sort of aerosol spray. As you spray it on the surface, some of it hits the target; most of it drifts away; and very little penetrates' (Mendelsohn 1968). Nevertheless, the view that the mass media can have a direct effect still has currency in some quarters.
- *Two-step model*: Katz and Lazarsfled (1955) suggested that the mass media work in stages. They argued that key opinion-leaders are active members of an audience who are influenced by the media. These opinion-leaders then transmit the messages to other people through personalized means of communication.
- *Uses and gratifications*: this theory posits that people interpret messages in accordance with 'wish fulfilment', i.e. 'people use the media to gratify their desires and satisfy their prejudices' (Tones and Green 2004). Berger (1991 cited in Tones and Green 2004) provides some examples of typical gratifications provided by the media and includes examples such as to be amused, to see authority figures exalted or deflated and to believe in romantic love.
- *Cultural effects model*: this model acknowledges the importance of social groups and communities. The media addresses people not as individuals but as members of identifiable groups, and media content is filtered and interpreted through cultural norms.

Features of effective interventions

Randolph and Viswanath (2004) in a review of the literature on mass media campaigns identified 'a set of factors or conditions that appear to contribute to the success of a campaign'. Their review draws principally on American studies; here you will learn about the features they identify as a framework to explore the use of the mass media in health promotion, taking an international perspective.

Getting the message across is the primary aim in mass communication interventions. This is conventionally achieved by buying media space or having it donated. Organisations such as the BBC World Service Trust has developed a different approach through working in partnership with national broadcasters, as illustrated by Ray Head in the following extracts.

 ### Size matters ... the world's largest-ever leprosy campaign

Leprosy is curable and the drugs are free. The missing link is that people don't know that. It was an issue that was crying out for an awareness campaign, particularly in India, where 60% of the world's leprosy cases are located.

Between 1999 and 2001 the British government (DFID) gave us more money than had ever previously been given for leprosy awareness: £1.1 million. For our funders it was a test case: could media campaigns really make the impact that we claimed were possible?

Our plans depended on one crucial variable: local ownership. Even with £1.1m we couldn't afford the huge quantities of airtime that would be needed to make the impact we wanted. We needed free airtime, on a massive scale, and the only way India's national media would give us that was if it became *their* campaign.

And so, over one year, my colleagues Peter Gill and Lori McDougall trained, coaxed and cajoled, drawing extraordinary creativity out of two government bureaucracies, Doordarshan TV and All-India Radio. It was a barter arrangement: we provided training, they did the production. And it took place on a gargantuan scale, working across five states in 20 languages, producing 37 TV advertisements and short dramas and 140 radio spots.

The films and spots were broadcast some 1500 times on Indian TV and 6000 times on All-India Radio, far more than we had been promised, and all free of charge. Worth £1.2m, this was a clear demonstration of the importance of local ownership. That same principle also applied to the medical side of the equation: our role was purely demand-creation, and it was crucial to have a close partnership with the Ministry of Health who would supply the actual treatment.

The impact of the campaign was much greater than we had anticipated. Over two campaign periods, some 200 000 people were positively diagnosed and treated for leprosy. And the stigma – a huge barrier to treatment in a country where leprosy is seen as hereditary and a curse of God – was dramatically reduced:

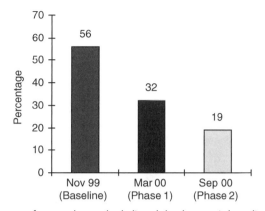

Figure 8.1 Percentage of respondents who believed that leprosy is hereditary

Source: 3 KAP surveys conducted by ORG Centre for Social Research in five states. Each sample size 1000, randomized. Subject to a sampling error of +/- 4% at the 95% confidence level.

Out of a target population of 458 million (the population of north India) the results in Figure 8.1 suggest that some 172 million people changed their minds about an issue that had been deeply ingrained for centuries.

But was it the *quality* or the *quantity* of the work which made this campaign such a success? We were able to measure the films' quality by extensive use of focus groups, yet these showed no correlation at all with the impact on attitudes and reported behaviours, which varied across different states. By contrast, there was an almost exact correlation between the level of impact in a given state, and the number of transmissions in that state (which did vary significantly). The power of volume and repetition – which was enabled by local ownership – were without doubt the decisive factor in the campaign's success.

Influencing the information environment and maximizing exposure

Mass media approaches are often supplemented with other means of transmitting messages such as the distribution of health education materials or the generation of news coverage in the 'free media', that is, the newspapers, magazines, TV and radio which are not paid for from the public pocket.

The cost of mass media interventions and the difficulty in sustaining them are two factors often raised as disadvantages of the approach. It is true that mass media campaigns can be extremely expensive (especially if you have to buy media space) and that for many campaigns the high impact achieved can not be sustained, but this is not always the case, as illustrated by Roy Head in the following extract.

 Small is sustainable: the phone-in show

In 1998, the UN Fund for Population Activities asked the BBC to set up an advertising campaign covering teenage sexual health issues in Vietnam. I'm a fan of advertising, in my opinion there's no better way of getting a message across than by high repetition, entertaining spots. But it struck me that Vietnamese youth had been talked *at* for 20 years. Wasn't it their turn to have a voice? So I persuaded UNFPA that a radio phone-in, where

Vietnamese youth could express their own questions and worries, would make a more dramatic impact. In its own way, it could even be a democratising influence.

Convincing the communist authorities was more of a challenge. There had never been a national phone-in in Vietnam, let alone one on sexual matters. So we invited 12 senior party officials to London to see the BBC's interactive programming. To my horror they were even given a guided tour of politicians being grilled on the BBC's *Newsnight* programme. To their credit, the Vietnamese decided that these were media skills they didn't have, and which – given the rise of AIDS and other youth problems – they now needed to learn.

I learnt a very important lesson next. We agreed with the authorities that the Youth Union would produce the programme for Voice of Vietnam Radio, using a presenter and two experts. I had envisaged recruiting a star-quality presenter, someone who would bring in a whole new sound and charisma. The Youth Union were outraged; in an emotional midnight phone call to the project manager, Julia Bicknell, they insisted that we were there to train *them*, not to recruit stars. Julia defied my instructions and agreed to work with their presenter, Thanh Van (below). She was right, I was wrong. That single decision, meaning that the show was fully integrated with their own programming and staffing, meant that they really *owned* it. And they were motivated to keep it going for some seven years after we left it in 1998. To this day it is the most sustainable project I have ever been a part of.

The other reason it was sustainable is because radio phone-ins are so *cheap*. The entire project, including all equipment and our management, cost just $80K. Once you've installed the telephone lines and a switcher to allow you to preview calls, the entire show runs for funds which are affordable in any country. Stations have to fill up airtime anyway, and this sort of interactive programme allows them to transform the 'feel' of the station. And with the same studio, they can invite their audience to talk about health, parenting, farming and even politics. The format is a perfect vehicle for development-oriented projects.

Finally we had to wait to see if – for the first time in their history – Vietnamese youth would call a national radio show and speak about their personal problems. The answer came in the very first call: 'I have HIV and I want to commit suicide'. Over the first 30 programmes there were no less than 4000 calls and 30 000 letters. Vietnamese youth had started to speak. And as I write, more than 7 years later, they're still talking.

Creative marketing, messages and message effects

While getting the message across might be considered the primary aim in mass communication interventions, getting the message *right* must be considered as equally important.

'Message framing' involves deciding between gain-framing versus loss-framing. Rothman *et al.* (cited in Randolph and Viswanath 2004) suggest that gain-framed messages were more effective in promoting prevention, whereas loss-framed messages were more effective in promotion early detection. The use of emotion is relevant in this context, and here the choice is most commonly between using negative emotions such as fear, and more positive ones, such as humour.

Supportive environments

For a campaign to be successful the environment must be such that individuals are able to make the changes called for. Randolph and Viswanath (2004) point to the reciprocal relationship between structural changes and media coverage: 'Media attention can strengthen the supportive environment for forming community coalitions and also lend legitimacy for policy and environmental change'.

 Activity 8.3

An explicit objective of many mass media campaigns is to influence the social context and to create a favourable climate in which interventions can be received. Think how this might come about.

 Feedback

A college principal/bar owner/garage owner is not sure if it was appropriate to install a condom machine in his sixth form college/bar/garage. He feels reassured and validated by a government-backed mass media campaign promoting condom use. A young person, motivated to use condoms by the same campaign, is further encouraged to do so because they are readily available in the college/bar/garage in which he studies/drinks/buys petrol. This is known in the USA as 'diffusion acceleration'.

It is difficult to assess the distinct contribution of different components of a campaign, but it is important to address this in evaluation research. Preventive interventions are often designed on the assumption that we are working with a 'blank slate' – that there are no other influences on people's behaviour. Yet, health communication is much more than what goes on in a health promotion intervention. As you have learnt in earlier chapters, there are numerous influences on our behaviour. These are just as likely to contradict, as they are to be in harmony with, health advice. It is important to recognize that the biggest changes in behaviour, and therefore in health status, are likely to come about through forces other than health promotion interventions.

Theory-based campaigns

Theories are helpful both in creating appropriate message strategies and in choosing the right vehicles in which to place messages. Communication strategies are commonly based on models and theories derived from the behavioural sciences. Taken together these models highlight:

- the importance of knowledge and beliefs about health;
- the importance of self-efficacy: the belief in one's competency to take action;
- the importance of perceived social norms and social influences related to the value an individual places on social approval or acceptance by different social groups;
- the importance of recognizing that individuals in a population may be at different stages of change at any one time;

- limitations to psychosocial theories which do not adequately take account of socioeconomic and environmental conditions;
- the importance of shaping or changing the environment or people's perception of the environment (Nutbeam and Hams 2004).

Such theories, it is suggested, 'are predicated on Western notions of individual autonomy and purpose' and 'may hold less relevance for populations in traditional communal cultures, where individual identity is grounded in family and community roles' (Elder 2001). UNAIDS developed a new framework for HIV/AIDS communication, which places a greater emphasis on the social and environmental context, as opposed to individual behaviour. It identified five domains of context as 'virtually universal factors in communications for HIV/AIDS preventive health behaviour', namely: government policy; socioeconomic status; culture; gender relations; and spirituality. Individual health behaviour is seen as a component of these domains, rather than the primary focus of health behaviour change (UNAIDS 1999).

Randolph and Viswanath (2004) identify a further feature relating to process analysis and exposure which you will consider in the next section on evaluation.

Evaluation

The major strength of the mass media – their ability to reach a wide audience – paradoxically also presents the greatest challenge for evaluation. Mass media interventions are less easily controlled than targeted interventions. In addition, there is less control over who receives the messages conveyed by the mass media, and how well the messages are understood. You need to be aware of three factors here:

- messages may fail to reach the audiences for which they were intended;
- messages may reach audiences for which they were not intended;
- messages may be misunderstood.

Mass media interventions may also have unintended consequences, over which health promotion agencies have little control. Further, as you will learn in Chapter 13, it has been suggested that provision of health information in this way may actually risk increasing health inequalities as it is argued that the generally better educated middle classes in a population are likely to benefit more.

Formative evaluation

Formative research uses exploratory work to guide the design of an intervention. An important component of formative research is the pre-testing of messages and materials. Pre-testing provides the opportunity to correct or modify messages. In turn, this ensures that messages are less likely to be misunderstood and misinterpreted.

Formative research typically uses focus groups to gauge whether:

- the tone and style of the materials are appropriate;
- they appeal to the target group;

- the information supplied, and the agency providing it, are seen as credible and authoritative;
- messages are understandable, relevant and realistic.

Information on the reading, listening and viewing habits of the target audience is also needed to ensure the appropriate channels are selected.

Another important goal of the formative phase of evaluation is to anticipate possible unforeseen outcomes. Often, these may well be favourable but may also be unfavourable. There are examples of mass media campaigns which have had the required beneficial effect on the target group, but have inadvertently had an adverse effect on other groups in the community (Wellings and Macdowall 2004).

Process evaluation

Process evaluation is undertaken while the intervention is running. This aims to answer two questions:

- Is the intervention succeeding or failing?
- What social and other factors are having an impact on delivery of the intervention which might be leading to success or failure?

Research should be capable of revealing not only *whether or not* a campaign has succeeded, but *why*. This allows findings to be used to guide future developments.

Exposure measures are a minimum requirement for process evaluation. There is also a need for more sophisticated process evaluation which sheds light on how and why an intervention succeeds or fails to achieve its goals. While outcome evaluation focuses on the extent to which the goals of a particular programme have been met, process evaluation is needed to provide insights into what factors may help or hinder their achievement.

By definition and design, exposure to the mass media is universal and it is difficult to tailor messages to specific target groups. In addition, problems of social and political acceptance can arise where messages are seen by those for whom they were not intended.

Specific issues to be addressed in process evaluation include the following questions:

- How well were resources allocated and disseminated?
- Did the intervention lead to any adverse side-effects?
- Was there harmony between the aims of health promotion and the needs of clients?
- Were there any social or political dynamics that interfered with the ways in which messages were received and responded to?
- Did the intervention interact with other interventions, or with environmental factors, to enhance the outcome?

Outcome evaluation

Important initial questions for outcome evaluation are:

- How can we measure success?
- How can we tell whether the effects can be attributed to the intervention?

In relation to both questions, there are aspects of mass media work which are problematic for evaluation.

Observed effects will be small

Broad spectrum interventions do not target high-risk individuals who have greater scope for change. Achieved change at the large and undifferentiated population level is therefore likely to be smaller. This may lead to criticism that campaigns have not achieved their objectives.

It is difficult to attribute effects to mass media intervention

Attributing outcomes to a specific intervention is difficult where mass communication techniques are used. An effective campaign will have an effect far beyond its original remit by creating media discussion by providing the impetus for local efforts, and so on. This means that it is not easy to separate the effects of the intervention from the effects of other events which are either running parallel with it or which are triggered by it.

A vital question in outcome evaluation relates to how large the effect has to be in order to say that the intervention has worked. Gains made in the case of mass media interventions may be modest because of the following four factors:

- *The size of the target population*: effects will be smaller where the target group is large and heterogeneous.
- *The nature of outcome measures or endpoints*: changes may be small because the wrong level of objectives has been chosen. Where measures of morbidity and mortality are used as outcomes in interventions aimed at the general population, unless the sample is impossibly large, the scale of the effect may be small and so seen to represent a failure of the intervention.
- *The scope of the intervention*: observed effects may be small because the endpoints are too narrowly conceived in terms of individual behaviour and do not take sufficient account of the social context.
- *The time scale*: the time scale looked at may be too short. Health promotion interventions may not show significant effects for some time.

A major challenge in assessing efficacy is how to attribute an outcome to an intervention. This is made harder in the case of mass communication interventions by the problem of 'background noise' (influences on the target audience other than the intervention). We need to ask three questions here:

- How can we be sure that the effects seen are truly the outcome of public education campaigns?
- How can we be sure that they are not the result of already existing differences?
- How can we be sure that the effects are not the result of exposure to something other than the intervention (such as the mass media generally or local preventive interventions)?

Where mass media interventions work well, it is likely to be (a) because they activate a complex process of change in social norms and (b) because they have a direct impact on individual behaviour. The evidence is that interventions with several components seem to work better than those with only one. A valid goal for an intervention may be to accelerate behaviour trends that already exist, rather than initiating new trends.

'Background noise' – often considered problematic in the context of outcome evaluation – also has the potential to provide continuity and reinforcement to mass media campaigns. Seen in this way, the task of outcome evaluation is to look at the extent to which a mass media intervention is successful in using environmental influences to achieve its own ends.

Outcome measures are determined by the objectives of the intervention. Lack of clarity over the scope of objectives of mass media interventions is a common problem for evaluation. It is not always clear, for example, to what extent it has been an explicit objective of mass media campaigns to modify individual behaviour and to what extent it has been to influence the social environment. Setting objectives at an inappropriate level can threaten the apparent success of the intervention.

Careful thought is therefore needed on what should count as reliable outcomes. In most cases, the immediate outcome variables will be the adoption and main-tenance of behaviours that reduce risk. These, rather than the more distal outcomes such as incidence of disease, morbidity or mortality, may constitute the indicators themselves, an example being condom use.

Summary

You have seen how using the mass media in health promotion has both strengths and weaknesses. This had led to a reassessment of the media's potential and limitations. The strength of the mass media, according to some, lies in helping to put issues on the public agenda, in reinforcing local efforts, in raising conscious-ness about health issues and in conveying simple information. The mass media are less effective in conveying complex information, teaching skills, shifting attitudes and beliefs, and changing behaviour in the absence of other enabling factors.

It is certainly true that in some cases the use of the mass media may be less effective than face-to-face methods of addressing target groups. Yet radio, television, news-papers and magazines are important sources of health information. You can't reach everyone through community approaches – and high-profile communication can reach hidden groups in the general population.

References

Elder JP (2001) *Behaviour Change & Public Health in the Developing World*. Thousand Oaks, CA: Sage.

Escobar-Chaves SL, Tortolero SR, Markham CM, Low BJ, Eitel P, Thickstun P (2005) Impact of the media on adolescent sexual attitudes and behaviours. *Paediatrics*, 116: 303–26.

Finnegan JR Jr, Viswanath K (1997) Communication theory and health behavior change, in K. Glanz, FM Lewis, BK Rimer (eds) *Health Behaviour and Health Education*, 2nd edn. San Francisco: Jossey-Bass.

Katz E, Lazarsfeld P (1955). Personal influence. New York: The Free Press.

Mendelsohn H (1968) Which shall it be? Mass education or mass persuasion for health? *American Journal of Public Health*, 58: 131–7.

Naido J, Wills J (1994) *Health Promotion Foundations for Practice*. London: Baillière Tindall.

Nutbeam D, Harris E (2004). Theory in a nutshell (2nd edition) Sydney: McGraw-Hill.

Randolph W, Viswanath K (2004) Lessons learnt from public health mass media campaigns: marketing health in a crowded media world. *Annual Review of Health*, 25: 419–37.

Tones K, Green J (2004) Mass communication and community action, in *Health Promotion Planning and Strategies*, London: Sage.

UNAIDS/Penn state (1999) Communications framework for HIV/AIDS. A new direction. Switzerland: UNAIDS.

Wellings K, Macdowall W (2000) Evaluating mass media approaches, in; Coombes Y, Thorogood M (eds), Evaluation of health promotion (2nd edition). Oxford: Oxford University Press.

9 Media advocacy

Overview

In this chapter you will learn about media advocacy as a strategy for public health policy change. You will be introduced to the key features and concepts in media advocacy and will consider how it differs from other approaches, such as lobbying, public relations and social marketing. Finally, you will consider the evidence for its effectiveness and the challenges it poses for evaluation.

Learning objectives

After reading this chapter, you will be better able to:

- explain the principles and key concepts of media advocacy
- describe public health contexts in which media advocacy can be applied
- explain the strategic issues involved in the use of media advocacy
- describe how media advocacy differs from other approaches to health promotion
- describe the issues that media advocacy presents for evaluation

Key terms

Agenda-setting Process by which the media influence what the public and policy makers perceive to be important.

Creative epidemiology Presenting statistics in ways that make them more meaningful to the media and the public.

Framing How an issue is presented in the media.

Media advocacy The strategic use of mass media as a resource for advancing a social or public policy initiative.

What is media advocacy?

Media advocacy involves generating news media coverage of public health issues in order to highlight particular problems and advocate *policy* solutions. It is often undertaken as part of a broader programme of activities which might also involve campaigning, lobbying and community development. Media advocacy is often described as an 'upstream' approach, as it seeks to produce changes at societal and policy levels rather than at the level of individual behaviour. It is also conceived as a bottom-up grassroots approach, involving community mobilization and capacity-building, although there is less consensus on this element.

Media advocacy arose from a recognition that the mass media can play a significant role in public health. As you learnt in the previous chapter, the mass media are a powerful force for increasing public awareness of health issues and for changing attitudes and norms. The media can also confer status and legitimacy on invisible or taboo issues so that it becomes more acceptable to discuss them in public, and they can contribute to legislative change by influencing policy-makers' perceptions of a problem and exerting pressure for action.

At the same time, the mass media are often considered a detrimental force for public health. They can undermine efforts to improve health, by providing inaccurate and misleading information, glamourizing unhealthy behaviours and promoting health-damaging products. They may also perpetuate stereotypes of particular types of illness or disseminate a view of the causes of ill health which overemphasizes individual responsibility and neglects the role of social and economic factors (Wallack 1990). While this has led to ambivalence about the use of the media among some health promoters, others argue that, whatever their shortcomings, the media are too powerful a force to be ignored by those who seek to change society. It is argued that having your issue covered in the news media is nearly always a necessary precursor to effecting change (Chapman and Wakefield 2001). The challenge is to harness the powerful influence of the media in the service of, not against, public health goals.

How do the media influence public health policy?

The media influence policy through a process called 'agenda-setting'. This concept, identified in the 1960s by communication scientists, refers to the process by which the media influence what the public and policy-makers perceive to be important. Agenda-setting can work in a number of different ways. Media coverage can raise awareness of a hitherto 'invisible' issue, or it can heighten existing public concern. In turn, this combined media and public attention can put an issue on the policy agenda and, through real or perceived pressure on policy-makers, can compel them to take action. One example is the 'discovery' of child abuse as a social problem in the USA. In 1962 a medical journal article reported on the rise in cases of 'battered child syndrome'. Broadsheet newspapers and television picked up on the story because it was 'newsworthy'; the subject was new, shocking and emotionally engaging. Sustained media pressure over several years led policy-makers first to recognize that this was an important social problem, and then to take legislative and policy action to protect children. Sometimes media coverage responds to rather than leads public opinion, and often the two interact; the media may pick up on an issue of concern to a minority section of the public, and report it in such a way that other sections of the public revise their initial opposition or indifference, leading to a groundswell in public opinion which itself becomes newsworthy.

Agenda-setting contributes to changes in policy because policy-makers are sensitive to what they perceive as public opinion (as depicted through the media). The task for the media advocate is to use the media to shape how a problem is seen, so that the policy-making body perceives a demand from the public for a particular policy change or certain policy decisions become more acceptable to the population. Policy-makers themselves also attempt to set the agenda through the media, using them to foster a 'climate of public readiness' for potentially unpopular policies such as legislation on smoking in public places. Of course, public opinion and policy formation are complex processes, and many other factors come to bear besides the media. Nevertheless, the belief that the media are a key agent in the policy process underpins media advocacy.

History of media advocacy

Media advocacy evolved as a concept in the 1980s in the USA, when tobacco control activists began arguing that they needed to be more skilled in gaining access to the media in ways that contributed to the adoption of smoking control policies. By this, they meant using attention-grabbing techniques to generate news coverage which would make the case for restrictions on tobacco marketing and on smoking in public places. In the early 1990s, alcohol campaign groups followed suit, as did public health practitioners and tobacco control researchers in Australia and New Zealand (Chapman and Lupton 1994). Academic interest in media advocacy grew during the early 1990s, and a number of papers were published describing the principles of the new approach and attempting to assess whether it was effective. Various 'activist toolkits' started to appear, first in print and later on the internet.

Media advocacy has been used most widely in tobacco control and, to a lesser extent, alcohol campaigns, although it has been applied to many different health issues, including: food content and labelling; gun control; location of mobile phone transmitters; swimming pool safety; the removal of lead water pipes from public housing; the use of imagery which might encourage violence against women; and legislation and stricter enforcement on drink-driving (Stead *et al.* 2002).

 Activity 9.1

Think of a story which you read in the press, which you think might have influenced public or government opinion about an issue, or which could influence opinion in the future. Why do you think that the story was influential?

 Feedback

You should have thought about issues such as: how the story was covered (what sort of messages); how long it was in the news; and how different people (including policy-makers) responded to it.

Defining features of media advocacy

There are three defining features of media advocacy, as follows.

Using the news media

The news media are seen to be more credible and authoritative than paid advertising, and to provide greater scope for complex policy debates. However, paid advertising might be used as part of a media advocacy intervention; deliberately shocking advertising, for example, is one way of generating news.

Policy change not individual behaviour change

The aim of media advocacy is to influence the social and economic determinants of public health issues rather than to change individual behaviour. Media advocacy does this through influencing those policies which shape the structural environment. These may be, for example, policies which regulate the activities of health-damaging industries, or policies governing the level of resources to be allocated to an issue.

Community organization

Wallack *et al.* (1999) define media advocacy as 'the strategic use of news media, and, when appropriate, paid advertising, *to support community organizing* to advance a public policy initiative' (emphasis added). They argue that media advocacy should be 'rooted in the needs of the community' and should seek to build the community's capacity to make its views represented in the media. This might involve working with the community to form pressure groups or coalitions, or the provision of training in media skills and advocacy to community workers and volunteers. Where media advocacy initiatives do this, they may be more sustainable and have wider benefits, such as increased community empowerment.

In practice, the community dimension is often not emphasized. Many media advocacy initiatives have been led by what could be termed public health 'elites' (such as medical associations or health authorities) rather than by community groups. Wallack *et al.*'s (1993) argument raises the question of how 'the community' is defined. As you will learn in Chapter 11, 'community' defies simple definition. A 'community' most often relates to a geographical area (such as a village) – but such a community is not homogenous. It is made up of people of different ages, ethnicities, interests and aspirations, some of which will conflict. In addition, some groups within the community may oppose measures which public health professionals believe to be in the community's best interest, such as fluoridation of water supplies and immunization.

When is media advocacy a useful public health approach?

Media advocacy's concern with policy solutions to public health problems means that it lends itself more suitably to some issues than others. It is most appropriately used where there is a clear policy solution and where the policy environment surrounding the issue is contested; that is, where opposing forces have a financial or other interest in preventing the policy change (such as the tobacco or alcohol industries). Media advocacy is a less relevant strategy for tackling health problems where the solution is not primarily a policy one or where there is already a strong public consensus on what should be done.

Activity 9.2

Which of these could be defined as media advocacy, and why?

1 Some parents are concerned about the speed at which cars drive past the local school. They invite the local newspaper to a protest in which they hold up placards showing the number of recent accidents at that spot.
2 A polio eradication campaign group issues a news release highlighting the number of polio cases in central Africa in 2004.
3 Breast Cancer Awareness Week.
4 A director of public health issues a news release calling on the local water company to fluoridate the water.
5 A local environmental campaign group offers media training to local groups wanting to oppose water fluoridation.

Feedback

Not all campaigns which use the media could be described as media advocacy. There needs to be a clear policy objective, such as changing legislation or having more money spent on a problem. Both official bodies and campaign groups can use media advocacy, sometimes for opposing goals. Media advocacy may be used by both 'sides' in the same campaign.

Roots and close relations of media advocacy

Media advocacy shares features with several other approaches to health and social change. Figure 9.1 illustrates what might be considered some of media advocacy's key 'roots and relations'.

From *health promotion*, media advocacy derives its concern with public health goals and their structural and policy determinants, as well as an interest in different ways of using the mass media to influence health. As you have already learnt, some of the theory underpinning media advocacy, such as agenda-setting and also 'framing' (see 'Doing media advocacy' below), originates in *communication science*.

Media advocacy shares elements with *social marketing* (see Chapter 10). Both are strategic approaches to social change which involve objective-setting, targeting,

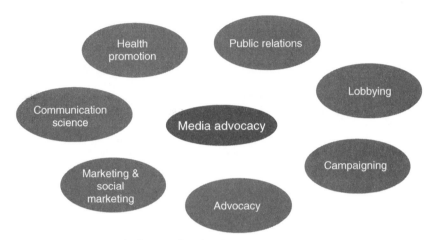

Figure 9.1 The roots and relations of media advocacy

the use of research, a communications mix and attention to message design. Some proponents of media advocacy have, however, argued that fundamental differences exist between the two approaches. Wallack (1990) has argued that social marketing is too individually focused and neglects the wider determinants of health. Social marketers, however, tend to be more pluralistic, regarding media advocacy as one possible strategy to be used in tandem with, or as part of, a social marketing approach. Contrary to Wallack's view, social marketers also argue that social marketing is as much concerned with changing the behaviour of groups, organizations and societies as it is with individual behaviour (see Chapter 10).

Media advocacy clearly draws on the broader concept of *advocacy*, of which it could be considered a subset. Advocacy involves supporting or arguing in favour of a cause, policy or idea. It can include speaking out on behalf of disadvantaged groups, tackling stigma and lobbying for policy improvements. It can also be undertaken to influence public opinion and societal attitudes or to bring about changes in government, community or institutional policies.

A key contributor to media advocacy's development was the growth in international consumer activism and *campaigning*. Publicity around the international boycott of Nestlé, for its intensive marketing of powdered milk in developing countries, can be seen as an early example of media advocacy. Media advocacy tactics are akin to those used by environmental pressure groups who seek to highlight governmental and corporate culpability for environmental problems and to argue for policy-level solutions. Similar tactics are used in the fields of housing, mental health and HIV/AIDS. It could be argued that pressure groups had been 'doing media advocacy' a long time before the concept was articulated within the public health movement.

The last two of media advocacy's 'roots and relations' are *lobbying* and *public relations*. Although lobbying often refers to 'behind the scenes' communication with law-makers to influence the legislative process, there is also a more public-faced, mass media-oriented form of lobbying which shares elements with media advocacy. Called 'outside' lobbying, this involves mobilizing members of the general public to exert pressure on officials within the policy-making community or communicating aspects of public opinion to policy-makers in order to demonstrate that an issue is of wide social concern.

Public relations relies on a sophisticated understanding of communication techniques, message development, segmentation and targeting, relationship-building and the use of research to inform all aspects of the communication process; concepts which are all relevant to media advocacy. However, public relations is primarily concerned with maintaining the reputation of the client, while media advocacy is usually conducted to advance a particular policy goal. Some proponents of media advocacy feel that it has an ethical dimension which is absent from public relations (which is often harnessed in the service of organizations and causes considered antithetical to public health, such as the tobacco and food industries). Others, however, argue that the two approaches are in practice very similar.

 Activity 9.3

Some people have argued that there is little new in media advocacy – it is simply a new label to describe an activity in which both the public health community and people outside it have been engaged for many years. What do you think?

 Feedback

Media advocacy derives aims, strategies, values and tactics from a wide range of disciplines and approaches. Its defining features are that it uses the news media to advocate policy solutions to public health issues and, according to some, should be community-led. It is concerned with the wider determinants of health and arguably has an ethical dimension. These features distinguish it from many of its roots and relations but there is some overlap.

Doing media advocacy

Media advocacy should not be seen as a 'magic bullet' and used in isolation, but rather as part of a process which may involve several different activities, in a programme of work designed to contribute to the overall policy goal. As with all approaches to health promotion, implementing media advocacy requires strategic thinking to maximize the chances of success. To develop a strategy you should answer five key questions:

* What is the problem?
* What is the solution?
* Who has the power to make the necessary changes?
* Who must be mobilized to apply pressure for change?
* What message would convince those with the power to act for change?

You also need to remember that the news media environment is unpredictable and constantly changing and you must be able to respond creatively and flexibly. The unpredictability of media advocacy initiatives also poses challenges for evaluation. Figure 9.2 is a framework for planning media advocacy.

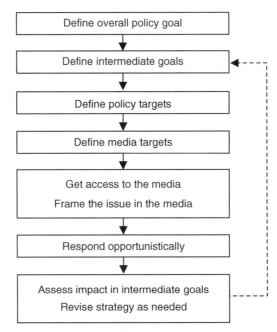

Figure 9.2 A framework for planning media advocacy

Define overall policy goal

Policy goals may include:

- persuading policy-makers of the need for a new policy;
- demanding more stringent enforcement of an existing policy;
- getting rid of or modifying a bad policy;
- encouraging policy-makers to stick with a good policy in the face of opposition.

'Raising awareness' or 'stimulating debate' about an issue are not policy goals, although they may be intermediate steps on the way to a policy goal.

Define intermediate goals

There may be a number of intermediate steps which can help prepare the ground for policy change. These might include increasing the frequency with which a topic is discussed in public or changing the language used to describe it. Other intermediate goals may include encouraging professional bodies to speak out or publish reports on the issue. Each of the intermediate goals may require different media advocacy activities, and the strategy should reflect this.

Define policy targets

This involves identifying who has the power to make the changes identified in the goals. The target can be a governmental body, a regulatory agency or an industry involved in harmful practices. It may be as narrow as an individual legislator, hospital manager or local retailer.

Define media targets

Different media outlets are appropriate for different goals. Getting an issue covered in the serious 'broadsheet' press will attract the notice of government ministers and civil servants, but if the aim is to convince policy-makers that there is wide-scale public indignation about a problem, the popular press may be more appropriate because its coverage tends to be more emotional and crusading. Policy-oriented stories are likely to appeal more to national news media, while 'human interest' stories which personalize the issue and seek to provoke strong emotions are likely to appeal more to tabloids, regional and local radio and 'women's magazines'.

Get access to the media

In order to generate news coverage, media advocates must 'gain access' to the news media and persuade them to cover a particular story. This requires media advocates to 'think like a journalist' and develop an understanding of what is 'newsworthy' and will appeal to a newspaper and its readers. Large newspapers receive hundreds of press releases a day, so media advocates need to make sure their stories stand out and are fresh. Newsworthy stories often involve controversy, conflict, injustice or irony. Other tactics include the use of interesting spokespeople such as celebrities or 'unlikely allies' (e.g. religious leaders speaking out in favour of condom use or gay rights). Media advocates frequently build a story around new research findings and major studies have often played an influential role in policy change. Research findings are rarely unequivocal and often need to be interpreted and packaged in a way which brings them to life for journalists and readers. A key concept which can help here is 'creative epidemiology' (Chapman and Lupton 1994) – the presentation of statistics in ways that make them more meaningful to the media and the public. Large numbers can be made more easily understood by putting them in a smaller local context. For example, rather than talking about the number of people diagnosed with a disease in a year, estimate the number in a day or an hour, or in a particular town. Another tactic is to make ironic comparisons, such as comparing the amount of money spent on advertising junk food with the amount spent on healthy eating campaigns.

Much effort is put into cultivating and nurturing relationships with key media professionals, as advocates are more likely to gain media access if they are known to individual journalists and can tailor their stories to the needs of these individuals.

Frame the issue in the media

Media advocates have to 'frame' their stories in a way that advances their objectives. It is important to frame a story so as to communicate clearly why this is a problem and that there is a specific policy solution. A story with the message 'childhood obesity is a multi-faceted problem and the solution is very complex' is neither newsworthy nor strategically useful; 'we need to ban commercial vending machines in school for a start' is, however, both. How a story is framed also influences where readers attribute responsibility for it.

 Activity 9.4

Compare how the following stories about women's drinking habits are framed. For both, try to identify who is responsible for the problem and what the policy solution is.

'More and more young women are drinking too much alcohol because they don't know the risks.'

'More and more young women are drinking too much because they're surrounded by powerful advertising and low price offers for alcohol.'

 Feedback

The first story portrays the women themselves as ignorant and irresponsible, while the second emphasizes that health is shaped by environmental factors too – in this case, the alcohol industry. It also makes clear that those who sell alcohol and those who regulate its sale also have a responsibility for solving the problem.

Framing is particularly important when media advocates face opposition from companies which sell harmful products.

 Activity 9.5

Think about the way that tobacco, alcohol and fast-food companies frame the smoking, drinking and eating of their products to make them seem attractive. How can media advocates frame these issues to create equally compelling public health arguments?

 Feedback

Tobacco companies frame smoking as an issue of individual choice in which heavy state intervention is unnecessary and inappropriate. Alcohol companies say that they should not be blamed if a small minority abuse their products; fast-food companies say that it is parents' responsibility to control what their children eat. These are powerful frames because they appeal to 'common sense' and chime with free market values. Media advocates need to respond with frames which are just as compelling. One powerful framing tactic is to depict health-damaging companies preying on vulnerable children with seductive messages. Not only do these stories have emotional appeal but they also undermine the companies' positioning of themselves as legitimate commercial enterprises.

Respond opportunistically

Where issues are debated in the media, the argument is likely to take many twists and turns. Any media advocacy initiative must be flexible enough to respond, which means being ready to counter statements by opponents and always looking for opportunities to create more news. One effective way of doing this is by 'piggybacking' onto breaking events and stories. The 2005 UK television series by celebrity chef Jamie Oliver, which exposed the 'scandal' of school meals, provided an excellent opportunity for nutrition campaigners to exploit the public concern and outrage generated by the programme.

Assess impact on intermediate goals and revise strategy as needed

Throughout the process, media advocates constantly assess progress towards their intermediate goals. Ongoing evaluation should be used to assess which tactics are working and which need modifying, and also to assess whether the goals themselves need changing.

Does media advocacy work?

Attempts to examine the effectiveness of media advocacy have relied in the most part on case study accounts, and more rarely on 'before-and-after' outcome evaluations. Case studies have tried to attribute media advocacy's contribution to a range of outcomes from national and regional legislation to cutting curbs on industry. Outcome evaluations have tended to measure intermediate outcomes, such as changes in media coverage or in specific actions (e.g. sales of age-restricted products). It is difficult to draw firm conclusions about effectiveness from these studies, and comparisons between different interventions is difficult because evaluation methods and measures vary widely. It is also difficult to attribute the specific contribution of media advocacy to changes at a policy level from other actions and influences.

Several studies suggest that media advocacy can influence the amount and type of news coverage given to a particular health issue. When implemented in conjunction with other activities, such as enforcement and community 'mobilization', it can also lead to policy changes, such as reductions in tobacco advertising in shops and alcohol sales to children. Case studies suggest that it has played an influential role in securing the passage of a number of pieces of legislation, mostly regarding tobacco and alcohol control, although these are often based on partial and anecdotal evidence. Not all media advocacy interventions have been effective. Two published examples are an Australian campaign about swimming pool fencing

(Chapman and Lupton 1994) and an initiative by the US group Mothers Against Drunk Driving to persuade Massachusetts to pass drink-driving legislation (DeJong 1996).

The Community Trials Project is one of very few studies which has attempted to estimate the contribution of media advocacy to health outcomes, in this case alcohol-related car crashes (Voas 1997; Voas *et al.* 1997). The study involved media advocacy training and extra resources for police enforcement to detect and deter drink-driving. A rigorous evaluation found that media coverage increased in the experimental communities, that public perception of the risk of being caught for drink-driving increased, and that these in turn were associated with less reported drink-driving and fewer crashes.

A number of features appear to enhance the design and implementation of media advocacy interventions. Media training and skilful use of targeting appear to increase media responsiveness to stories. Message framing seems to be particularly important in contested policy environments, and ongoing research with the public can help to identify powerful and appealing messages. Several media advocacy interventions have used the findings of prestigious research reports to gain media interest and confer legitimacy on an issue. Attention to how research is packaged and disseminated is therefore important. The literature suggests that controversial and adversarial approaches can work in some contexts but in others they may run the risk of losing support, both from the wider community and within the media advocacy organization itself. Similarly, the literature suggests that community mobilization may be relevant in some interventions but not others, and that media advocacy can be implemented both as a top-down and as a bottom-up strategy – each can be appropriate, depending on the context.

The challenge of evaluation

Media advocacy poses a number of challenges for evaluation. The range of activities defined as media advocacy, from unpaid publicity components of multi-component interventions to small-scale local activism, raises issues about what is being evaluated and, as you have learnt, media advocacy is often undertaken as part of a range of activities, so attributing any effects to the media advocacy element can also be problematic.

The randomized controlled trial (RCT), often regarded as the 'gold standard' of evaluation, may be difficult to apply to many media advocacy interventions. Media advocacy activities are 'fuzzy' interventions which are not easily described in terms of programmes (Chapman and Lupton 1994), and do not lend themselves to precise statement as independent variables whose effects can be measured. Furthermore, the experimental design is inappropriate for those initiatives which are unpredictable, which take place over a very long timescale, or which involve changes in tactics and actions. In addition, evaluation must examine process as well as outcomes. Evaluation should explore: the nature of the media coverage and how audiences interpreted it; the processes by which media advocacy efforts exert an influence on opinion-formers and policy-makers; and interventions' unexpected and/or indirect effects which may in themselves be deemed worthwhile, such as increases in community participation in the policy process or gradual shifts in community attitudes towards a health problem.

Evaluations of media advocacy can incorporate evaluation methods developed for the other fields on which media advocacy draws: communication and media studies, public relations, political campaigning, advocacy, social marketing and so forth. Finally they need to use multiple methods, both quantitative and qualitative; no one type of method is capable of capturing the complexity and multiple perspectives.

A framework for evaluating media advocacy interventions (Stead *et al.* 2002) proposes that formative, process and outcome evaluation are useful:

- Formative research can be used to guide overall strategy; for example, by exploring how policy-makers and the public perceive a particular issue and by gauging likely levels of support or opposition to a particular policy. Similarly, focus groups and pre-testing can help to design specific messages.
- Process evaluation is also important. While impact and outcome evaluation tell us whether or not an intervention succeeded, process evaluation can help to explain why it did or did not do so, by examining the factors which influence its implementation. Process evaluation can answer a number of questions specific to a media advocacy initiative such as:
  - What tactics and strategies were used by advocacy groups to reduce or cancel out the power of opposition groups?
  - How feasible and acceptable were different framing strategies?
  - How are public opinion and the public health actions of politicians related to each other?
  - What factors appear to encourage policy-makers and politicians to act on a public health issue?
  - What does it mean to say that some individuals are 'good' at media advocacy, and what can be learned from them?
- Outcome evaluation should examine five kinds of outcome:
  - 'Media outcomes' – the impact of the media advocacy initiative on the local media: what coverage was generated; how this coverage was framed; and how it was received by target-group audiences?
  - 'Public-opinion outcomes' – the impact of the coverage, and of accompanying media advocacy activities such as community organizing, on public perceptions of the public health issue in question.
  - 'Policy outcomes' – impacts on policy-makers and the policy process. If media advocacy seeks to influence conditions within the community that are deleterious to health and to increase the community's capacity to participate in actions to improve its health, then it is also appropriate to measure changes at this level.
  - 'Community capacity outcomes' – changes in community conditions and in community participation in health promotion actions.
  - 'Advocacy capacity outcomes' – changes in the skills and status of the media advocacy practitioner/organization, which, while they might have no direct bearing on the public health goal in question, increase the capacity of the practitioner/organization in the longer term.

Summary

Media advocacy is an approach for using the media in order to advance particular policy solutions. It originated within the tobacco and alcohol control movements in the 1980s. It has three key features: it uses the news (unpaid) media rather than advertising; it is concerned with policy change not individual behaviour change; and, according to some but not all proponents, it also includes grassroots community organization and capacity-building.

Media advocacy involves influencing how the news media cover public health stories. This is assumed to influence public opinion, which in turns leads to pressure on policy-makers to act. This is achieved through a process called 'agenda setting'.

It is difficult to draw firm conclusions on the effectiveness of media advocacy because interventions vary widely, as do evaluation methods. Furthermore, the specific contribution of media advocacy to changes at a policy level is difficult to disentangle from other actions and influences. However, there is evidence to suggest that media advocacy can influence the amount and type of news coverage given to a particular health issue. When implemented in conjunction with other activities, it may also lead to policy-level changes. Case study accounts suggest that it may have played an influential role in securing the passage of a number of pieces of legislation, mostly regarding tobacco and alcohol control.

The evaluation of media advocacy poses several challenges. RCTs are difficult to apply to many media advocacy interventions. Furthermore, on its own outcome evaluation will fail to capture some of the effects and processes which are of most interest. A multi-faceted approach to evaluation, which examines inputs and processes as well as impacts at media, public opinion, policy, community and organizational levels, is needed.

References

Chapman S, Lupton D (eds) (1994) *The Fight for Public Health: Principles and practice of media advocacy*. London: BMJ Publishing Group.

Chapman S, Wakefield M (2001). Tobacco control advocacy in Australia: reflections on 30 years of progress. *Health Education and Behavior*, 28(3): 274–89.

DeJong W (1996) MADD Massachusetts versus Senator Burke: a media advocacy case study. *Health Education Quarterly*, 23(3): 318–29.

Stead M, Hastings GB, Eadie D (2002) The challenge of evaluating complex interventions: a framework for evaluating media advocacy. *Health Education Research Theory and Practice*, 17(3): 351–64.

Voas RB (1997) Drinking and driving prevention in the community: program planning and implementation. *Addiction*, 92(S2): S201–19.

Voas RB, Holder HD, Gruenewald PJ (1997) The effect of drinking and driving interventions on alcohol-involved traffic crashes within a comprehensive community trial. *Addiction*, 92(S2): S221–36.

Wallack L (1990) Two approaches to health promotion in the mass media. *World Health Forum*, 11: 143–54.

Wallack L, Dorfman L, Jernigan D, Themba M (1993) *Media Advocacy and Public Health: Power for prevention*. Thousand Oaks, CA: Sage.

Wallack L, Woodruff K, Dorfman L, Diaz I (1999) *News for a Change: An advocate's guide to working with the media*. Thousand Oaks, CA: Sage.

10 | Social marketing

Overview

Social marketing takes ideas and techniques that are used in the commercial sector to influence consumer behaviour and applies them to health behaviour. The logic is that if the Philip Morris company is so successful in persuading young people to take up smoking, maybe we can learn from what they do and use similar approaches to dissuade young people from smoking. It also makes sense to learn more about marketing in order to control its effects in the hands of 'hazard merchants' like the tobacco and fast-food industries. This chapter therefore presents a series of discussions about the key principles of commercial marketing and how these might be applied in health promotion. It assumes no previous knowledge.

Learning objectives

After reading this chapter, you will be better able to:

- describe the basic principles of social marketing
- construct a basic marketing plan
- distinguish between social marketing and social advertising

Key terms

Competitive analysis Assessments of what competing organizations (such as the tobacco companies) are doing in order to inform efforts to control or compensate for these.

Consumer orientation Why people choose to do as they do – what ideas, emotions and aspirations influence them.

Customer-defined quality What the user thinks of an intervention or service.

Relationship marketing Action to build ongoing, mutually beneficial relationships with our target groups.

Stakeholder marketing Activities aiming to influence the behaviour of those groups who shape the social environment (e.g. policy-makers or health professionals).

Introduction

Forget everything you know about social marketing; everything you have read, heard or been told. In particular, forget any notion that social marketing is just some slightly tacky synonym for social advertising. We want to start with a blank sheet of paper and explain from first principles what social marketing is and why it is worth your while to get to know it better. We want to do this, not because social marketing is some sort of panacea or revolutionary super-solution, but because it can provide useful insights for health promoters in their attempts to influence human behaviour.

The most basic – and universally accepted – truth about social marketing is that it takes learning from commercial marketing and applies it to the social and health sectors (Kotler and Zaltman 1971). Ideas and techniques that are being used to influence consumer behaviour can cross the profit divide and be used to influence health behaviour. These ideas and techniques are extremely powerful. They underpin the unprecedented success of all major companies, from Nike to Philip Morris. They also explain why public health has been at such great pains to impose controls on the marketing of hazardous products such as tobacco, alcohol and fast food; and quite rightly too – recent reviews have shown that such marketing does influence our smoking, drinking and eating behaviours.

Australia, New Zealand, Canada and the US all have social marketing facilities embedded within their health services. In the UK, social marketing even reached the dizzy heights of being discussed in the government's White Paper on public health, which talks of the 'power of social marketing' and 'marketing tools applied to social good' being 'used to build public awareness and change behaviour' (Department of Health 2004).

The evidence base supports this interest: a recent systematic review shows that social marketing can deliver behaviour change, at least in the field of nutrition (McDermott *et al.* 2005). Of 25 good quality nutrition interventions found, 21 reported at least one statistically significant improvement in behaviour. So how do Nike do it, and what can we learn from them?

Marketing concepts and social marketing lessons

Consumer orientation

Marketing is based on a very simple idea: putting the consumer – rather than production – at the heart of the business process. While Henry Ford focused on selling what he could produce, offering his customer little choice but cheapness – 'any colour that he wants so long as it's black' – modern marketers invert this principle and produce what they can sell. This deceptively simple change has revolutionized commerce over the last 50 years, making Nike and Coca-Cola the giants that they are. It has succeeded because, paradoxically, listening to us consumers, putting us in the driving seat, actually makes it easier to influence our behaviour. This notion recognizes that our behaviour as consumers is *voluntary*. We can choose not to buy or to buy elsewhere. The market-place punishes those who forget this truth with oblivion.

Starting with the consumer means that marketers have to understand everything about us: what makes us tick; our hopes and dreams; our needs. They don't make assumptions or think they know best. Marketers also recognize that what seems obvious is often deceptive, and there is a corresponding need to think through what consumers really want.

Activity 10.1

In Browning's poem 'How they brought the good news from Ghent to Aix', three horse riders set out to deliver 'the news which alone could save Aix from her fate'. Two of their horses die during the gallop. Roland, our hero's horse, expires on the streets of Aix as the tidings are delivered. What was it the riders really needed?

Feedback

An acquisitive entrepreneur working in Ghent at the time might have tried to sell them better horses or even a motor bike. What they really needed – and any marketer worthy of the name would recognize this – was a telephone. They weren't looking for a means of transport at all, but a means of communication.

The point underlying this example is that consumers don't buy products, they buy solutions to problems. Marketers understand this and go to great lengths to divine our problems and provide ever more imaginative and intricate ways of solving them. In this way they seek, not to force us to buy, but to seduce us with mutually beneficial offerings.

Transposing this to public health, the danger from the social marketer's perspective is that we assume we know what people want: better health and longer life. It seems like a truism which is leant even greater credence by its evident worthiness. What people need, then, becomes a matter of professional judgement and rigorous epidemiology, followed by research on how these perfectly defined products can be sold to the public. So, like latter day Henry Fords, at best we offer people phoney choices, such as a European anti-smoking campaign which suggested that young people should 'feel free to say no' to tobacco. There is no freedom in such a choice. Evidence points to a more complex picture. Why would any of us smoke, drive racing cars, have unprotected sex or do any of the multiplicity of health-damaging things that we would never do if life were simply about minimizing risk and optimizing our physical health and longevity? We can't all be ignorant. Indeed survey after survey shows that we aren't. We know these things are dangerous, but we still do them. Our reasons are many and various: life is difficult and we need ways to cope with it – sometimes dysfunctional ways. We need to take risks to make things more interesting; we have to live with the fact of our own mortality.

Commercial marketers are all too ready to latch onto our anxieties and hopes. Elizabeth Arden offers beauty, Garnier youth and Pentax immortality. Social marketers don't advocate interventions involving cosmetics but they would suggest that a recognition of the complexities of life, and the need to help people navigate these, is integral to sustained behaviour change. We are in the empowerment business.

Activity 10.2

Think of any ways in which you have added additional, avoidable risk into your life in the last 12 months. You may have got involved in a sport which threatened injury, work that tested your abilities and ran the risk of causing embarrassment in front of your colleagues, or practised a new skill in public such as singing or playing a musical instrument. Not all these things endanger your physical health, nor are they undesirable – but they are risky. Now think for a moment about why we take such unnecessary risks.

Feedback

It soon becomes apparent that we seek more than health and safety in life. Social marketers recognize that failing to understand these subtleties can push us down the road towards being directive. When people don't do what we wish – quit smoking, drink sensibly – we get cross and blame them. Not recognizing the importance of risk-taking also feeds the delusion that there is such a thing as the universally ideal public health product.

Customer-defined quality

Inventing the world's most effective mousetrap may seem like a guaranteed route to business success. But your impending wealth will also depend on potential customers knowing about your new trap and being able to access and afford it. In addition, they will need to trust you to deliver on your promise. More fundamentally, however, they will have to agree that it is indeed a great mousetrap and their opinions on what a good mousetrap is – just as much its technical performance – will determine this. If, for example, your customers can't bear the thought of killing mice, no amount of technological wizardry will convince them to buy a lethal trap. The most ineffective humane alternative will be preferable; will be a better product.

This thinking has made 'consumer-defined quality' a prominent business concept in recent years. It's not that technical expertise has become devalued; just that focusing on technical performance alone is dangerous – as the demise of the British motorcycle industry famously shows. The Norton Commando motorcycle was technically superb, and indeed is still drooled over by aficionados, but it did not respond to consumer demand for cleaner, smaller and more reliable bikes. Japanese manufacturers did, which is why Kawasaki and Honda now rule British roads.

Social marketers argue that this thinking from consumer behaviour has to be applied with equal rigour to health behaviour. This is potentially challenging stuff in a field dominated by the 'medical model' and professional expertise, where rigorous scientific decision-making is prized. Nonetheless, social marketers argue that, in the world of behaviour change, the target group's opinion about an offering is as important as the clinician's.

Tobacco control experts who develop 'evidence-based' smoking cessation clinics that offer what science shows to be the best possible service might argue that this is the 'Rolls Royce', the 'gold standard' offering. The social marketer replies that Rolls Royce went bust and the gold standard was abandoned because people didn't respect it. In the world of voluntary behaviour, the customer's view will prevail.

Activity 10.3

How might the principle of customer-defined quality change the focus in health promotion interventions?

Feedback

Respecting the customer's definition of quality places much more importance on 'intermediate measures' of success. Customer satisfaction is an important impact measure in its own right. For example, a drugs prevention intervention that makes young people feel more confident and empowered in their drug-related choices and provides a valued support at a vulnerable time of their lives should be judged extremely worthwhile. Some would say this is a more important measure than whether or not the intervention has any impact on their drug-taking behaviour.

No man is an island

Marketers are also disciples of John Dunne. They recognize that we are social beings and that our individual actions are greatly influenced by our surroundings. The business community has long recognized that economic success is not only dependent on their consumer marketing but also on the macroeconomic environment within which the company operates.

Standard marketing texts typically divide this macro-environment into five forces: physical; economic; social; technological; and political/legal. Effective business planning includes careful monitoring of these forces. In many instances they are largely uncontrollable. Technological developments, for example, or physical geography, cannot be manipulated at will. However, companies still need to know about them so that they can decide how to respond to the threats and opportunities they present.

However, in other instances, such as in the case of litigation and public policy, there is at least the potential for business to exert influence. As Jobber (2001) points out, 'Close relationships with politicians are often cultivated by organizations both to monitor political moods and also to influence them'. Furthermore, in many instances government sees this influence as perfectly legitimate and actively seeks the advice of relevant business sectors before proceeding. The tobacco industry is widely known to be active in this area. As Jobber goes on to note: 'The cigarette industry, for example, has a vested interest in maintaining close ties with government to counter proposals from pressure groups'. It is worth reiterating that Jobber's is a standard business text; he has no particular interest in public health. Thus, the commercial sector's consumer marketing efforts are complemented by equally comprehensive 'stakeholder marketing' efforts. The principles are exactly the same, it's merely the identity of the customer that varies.

Social marketers therefore welcome the broadening of health education into health promotion and see health promoting schools, tobacco advertising bans and 'fat taxes' as encouraging evidence of this wider agenda in action. They would add that marketing ideas and techniques should be brought to bear on the task. In particular, they emphasize the need to understand the customer, whether they are a government minister or a lone parent, and offer them attractive deals.

Competitive analysis

For the marketer, the competition (typically other companies) is a crucial part of the macro-environment and there are limits to how far mutually beneficial exchange will get you. Sometimes you have simply to take on and try to destroy your adversary. Nike and Adidas, Burger King and McDonald's, Philip Morris and Imperial Tobacco are therefore fierce rivals; stock market ratings are the business equivalent of sports leagues; takeovers and company failures are the obvious results for the winners and losers in this jockeying for position. These peer-group competitive pressures combine with similar forces from regulatory bodies and public interest organizations.

These forces are not blind and thoughtless and require a managerial response. Companies therefore put great effort into understanding the behaviours of their competitors and other stakeholders so that they can control, influence or at least adapt to the competition.

Good competitive analysis, as with so much else in marketing, starts by looking at the world through the eyes of the customer. What products do they use to satisfy the same need? What do they buy instead? Who do they see as the competition? Are McDonald's customers switching between them and Burger King or KFC? Or between them and the cinema? How do their customers see the current obesity debate? Do they have any sympathy with those New Yorkers suing fast-food companies or support a ban on fast-food advertising?

This analytical process helps define competitors and can then be applied directly to them. The activities of Philip Morris will help inform Imperial Tobacco about how they stand in their customers' and stakeholders' eyes, the possibilities for the future and the pitfalls to avoid. Similarly, the activities of tobacco control will be of great interest. More than any other competitor, tobacco control threatens their future prosperity, attacking them in the media, bearing witness against them in the courts and promulgating ever tighter regulation. This confrontation is inevitable; the objectives of the tobacco industry and public health are fundamentally at odds.

Social marketers advocate exactly the same kind of competitive analysis as Lazer and Kelly's (1973) long established definition recommends:

Social marketing is concerned with the application of marketing knowledge, concepts, and techniques to enhance social as well as economic ends. It is also concerned with analysis of the social consequence of marketing policies, decisions and activities.

Health promoters need to put themselves mentally in the boardrooms of big business – especially of the companies dubbed the 'hazard merchants' – and ask what are they doing, thinking and planning.

Strategic thinking

From a business perspective, the ultimate aim of this competitive analysis is to gain sustainable competitive advantage, with the emphasis on sustainable. Above all else, studying your rivals informs your strategic planning. It helps define where you want to be, not just in the next year but the next decade. And this long-term vision is invaluable. Rumour has it that one Japanese car manufacturer is more than happy to show their competitors around their factory, and give them as much information as they want about their production methods. By the time they have copied them, their erstwhile host will have moved on, made improvements and left them far behind.

The emphasis on the long-term in business is perhaps most evocatively illustrated through branding. The Coca-Cola logo is nearly a 100 years old and the Nike 'swoosh' has been with us for over 30 years. For the social marketer, such longevity is rare indeed.

 Activity 10.4

What factors militate against health promoters developing a brand identity for their work?

 Feedback

The political context, funding systems and a culture demanding immediate and dramatic behaviour change militate against it. In Scotland, for example, the principal government agency charged with delivering health promotion has changed its identity no fewer than four times in the last 25 years. What hope then that individual campaigns will retain any consistency? Nonetheless, social marketing principles suggest that such long-term approaches are needed if sustained behaviour change is to be achieved. Furthermore, these approaches will need to be both multifaceted and empowering. Note that there is no clear evidence base to support this conclusion – no randomized controlled trial showing that long-term, multifaceted and empowering health campaigns work. Instead, the conclusion rests on observation of what is happening in the commercial world.

In this sense, it is a quintessentially social marketing conclusion, and illustrates one of the key contributions the discipline can make. The commercial sector is essentially an enormous and fabulously resourced laboratory for testing out new ways of influencing behaviour, driven by a commercial imperative which makes these experiments both pragmatic and productive. Social marketing enables us in public health to steal their findings.

Relationships nor transactions

Long-term thinking and sustainable progress have entered the core elements of marketing, moving the discipline on from a focus on transactions with customers and stakeholders to one of building relationships with them. The basic ideas underpinning the discipline were laid down in the 1950s and were based on research in the fast-moving consumer goods sector. Military metaphors such as 'campaigns' and 'targets' were used, and a set of tools, typically comprising the four Ps of promotion, pricing, place and product design were applied to deliver the crucial requirement of consumer satisfaction. Objectives had to be realistic, measurable and focused on sales and profits. Exchange theory gave this thinking some theoretical basis and placed the emphasis very clearly on successful, but typically ad hoc, transactions.

These ideas continued to dominate until the mid-1980s, when serious criticisms emerged from research done in the service (e.g. banks) and business-to-business (e.g. marketing between component manufacturers and car producers) sectors. In the first case, the focus on sales overlooked the crucial service industry construct of customer satisfaction. In business-to-business marketing, the mass, transactional assumptions in fast-moving consumer goods marketing conflicted with a day-to-day reality of long-term, cooperative alliances between buyers. A more continuous and sophisticated model was needed.

Business also became increasingly conscious that customer loyalty mattered. It is much more expensive to acquire new customers than keep existing ones. The emphasis began to shift from one-off transactions to ongoing relationships (Grönroos 1994). Companies started to think not just about immediate but long-term profitability. Indeed, individual transactions may lose money, provided the 'lifetime value' of the customer is positive. This has fundamental implications for the business function, greatly increasing the importance of customer service and satisfaction. A EIU survey conducted in 2001 suggests that this lesson has been well learnt. It showed that customer satisfaction is taking over from profitability as the prime determinant of performance-related pay (Richardson 2001).

Relationship-building requires an ever more intimate knowledge of the customer. Until recently such insights were only possible on a small scale – a buyer dealing with a couple of dozen suppliers, or a local pub, for instance. Information technology has changed all that. Data mining, mobile communications, vastly enhanced computers, opportunistic and endemic data-gathering all provide even the biggest operators with the potential to understand and respond sensitively to their customers.

There are many benefits to relationship marketing. If customers remain loyal then planning is much easier, pricing becomes less critical and the developing trust brings opportunities to sell new offerings. Relational thinking can also be applied to suppliers, retailers, competitors (through alliances), employees and other stakeholders.

For social marketers this suggests there are benefits to be gained if we move beyond what might be termed the 'intervention mentality', and instead think in terms of building long-term relationships with our customers. Experience, backed by well established theory (e.g. stages of change), tells us that health behaviour changes do not generally occur overnight. They involve a series of steps from initial contemplation through to reinforcement, a process that is both dynamic and precarious; the individual can regress or change heart at any point.

Furthermore, behaviour change has both emotional and rational drivers. We know, for example, that young people smoke despite their knowledge of the health consequences because it makes them feel adult and fashionable. It is this that explains the tobacco industry's huge – and extremely long-term – investment in evocative brands.

Finally, social marketing is founded on trust. It is not driven by profit but, at least ostensibly, a desire to benefit the target audience. It therefore has a very different, and perhaps morally higher, base than commercial marketing on which to build mutual respect with its customers. If commercial marketers can seriously argue that 'the presence of commitment and trust ... is central to successful relationship marketing, not power and its ability to condition others' (Morgan and Hunt 1994), then social marketers have to listen.

Accepting the logic of relational thinking has two important implications for successful social marketing:

- In line with the points made above about strategic thinking, longer timeframes are essential or, more radically, as in commerce, perhaps we should opt for an indefinite timeframe. The Ford Motor Company have been successful for nearly a 100 years. Their basic product, the car, has remained the same while design and performance have rapidly improved in careful response to consumer need on the one hand, and advancing technological knowhow on the other. In the UK, the National Health Service brand has flourished for 50 years and, although it is frequently reviewed and reorganized, few would advocate closing it down. Why shouldn't social marketing programmes have similar longevity?
- Related to this, we need a greater degree of faith in the idea that if we stick at health promotion we will get it right. In point of fact this doesn't require a big leap of faith. The evidence base is extensive. In short, we *do* know what works.

Furthermore, the move to relational thinking in marketing is acquiring its own momentum. As more companies move to this way of doing business – building trust and partnerships, emphasizing customer service and satisfaction and rewarding loyalty – those who ignore it will become increasingly isolated. The successful marketing techniques of the 1950s, using a selection of tools to do things to what was conceived of as a passive customer, simply will not work on an increasingly active and critical populace. This is as true for social as it is for commercial marketing.

Activity 10.5

Reflecting on what we have discussed so far, jot down what you think are the key principles of social marketing.

 Feedback

The key principles of social marketing are:

• we are concerned with *voluntary* behaviour change
• a customer-focus should drive our efforts
• social context matters, so stakeholders are also important targets
• long-term relationships matter more than ad hoc transactions
• competitive analysis matters
• strategic vision ensures we have enough length and breadth to our efforts

Social marketing planning

So far you have learnt about the ideas behind marketing. You will now move on to the practicalities. The core tool underlying any marketing effort is the marketing plan (see Figure 10.1). This addresses a number of basic questions:

• Where are we now, and where do we want to be (strategic analysis)?
• Who (segmentation and targeting) will we need to get to do what (objectives) if we are to get there?
• What is the best way of ensuring the target groups do as we wish (formulation of strategy)?
• How can we monitor progress (research)?

The plan is not a fixed document that will be followed slavishly through to completion and then a new one drawn up. It is an ongoing effort that is continually honed and refined. As noted above, the assumption in marketing is that we are broadly going in the right direction. The need is for steady, if careful and well monitored, progress. Of course, sometimes things go badly wrong, dramatic changes are needed and indeed companies go bust. Nonetheless, in general a culture of incremental learning and careful control works well. Social marketers argue that there is no reason why a similar approach should not be applied to health promotion.

The strategic analysis essentially looks at the macroeconomic factors discussed above and sets marketing performance against this. A 'SWOT' analysis for example might be conducted to map the marketing organization's internal strengths and weaknesses against external opportunities and threats. The aim is then to ensure that opportunities are exploited and threats avoided by harnessing the organization's strengths and minimizing its weaknesses. This provides strategic direction. For example, an analysis of dental health in a particular region may suggest that fluoridation presents the greatest opportunity for bringing improvements, is politically popular with the current government and is well within the professional

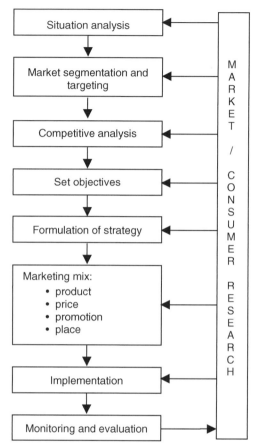

Figure 10.1 A social marketing plan

Source: Adapted from Hastings and Elliott (1993)

capabilities and capacity of the marketing organizations (Hastings *et al.* 2000). On the other hand, the only opposition comes from a vociferous but marginalized group of anti-fluoridationists.

Segmentation determines which group or groups might be able to help you make progress towards your aim. In the fluoridation example, it is clear that many groups are involved – including the media, politicians and the general public – but the water providers are the key players. The decision is therefore made to target all four groups, with the emphasis on the last. For the water companies, the objective is straightforward (if challenging): you want them to add fluoride to the public water supply.

The importance of competitive analysis to marketing has already been discussed. In this case the only serious opponents are the anti-fluoridationists. But they are implacable. No deals can be struck with them, no alignment of objectives is possible. Every effort therefore has to be made to limit their access to the media and undermine their credibility.

Marketing has traditionally been defined as a matter of 'getting the right product, at the right price, in the right place . . . presented in such a way as to successfully satisfy the needs of the consumer' (Cannon 1986). While noting what was said on relationship marketing, the formulation of strategy can be seen as the successful manipulation of these four Ps of product, place, price and promotion. Three points should be emphasized here. First, as always in marketing, the customer's view is pre-eminent. In Cannon's definition, 'right' means that it will best meet the customer's needs. Second, these four tools will be used collectively, each reinforcing and complementing the others. Indeed the four Ps are commonly known as the marketing mix. Third, note that advertising is only part of one of the Ps. This underlines the point made earlier: marketing and advertising are very far from being synonyms. Equating them is like equating mechanical engineering with the screwdriver.

In the fluoridation example, advertising would play a very small part; perhaps no more than the production of a leaflet to inform the public of your plans. Much more important would be to focus on the water providers and emphasize the benefits to them of fluoridation. Remember, private water companies are not interested in public health. They want – and indeed are legally required – to do just two things: provide their customers with clean water and their shareholders with a reasonable return. However, they may be interested in helping the government carry out its policies, retaining good relationships with public health professionals in their area and positive public relations. If framed correctly, fluoridation can provide all these benefits.

The monitoring of progress enables the marketer to retain some degree of control over events. Note, however, as illustrated in Figure 10.1, it is not an afterthought which kicks in when the strategy has been implemented, it is an ongoing process that guides decisions at every stage of the marketing plan. The next section looks in more detail at this marketing and consumer research process.

The role of research

Marketing calls for complex and continuous research with both consumers and stakeholders. At the same time, however, the market-place forces a degree of pragmatism. Decisions have to be made today, so perfect data tomorrow is of no use. There is also an acceptance that hunch and gut-feel will need to be brought to bear at least some of the time. Evidenced-based decision-making has a comforting ring at first, but it becomes slightly menacing when it gets in the way of manoeuvrability. Similarly, success is built gradually and continuously and is consequently ad hoc. We would argue that randomized controlled trials (RCTs), however high quality, are expensive and time-consuming and therefore have limited value; it doesn't help you to know – however precisely – what you should have done three years after the advertising campaign, product launch or rebranding exercise has finished. All this meshes neatly with the marketer's commitment to strategic thinking and relationship-building.

Social marketers welcome a flexible approach to research. They see it as a means of learning about their customers and stakeholders and hence providing a firm foundation for their strategic planning.

Summary

In this chapter you have learnt how social marketing has become so powerful, and demonstrated that concepts such as consumer orientation, stakeholder marketing, strategic planning and relationship-building can be used to influence health as well as consumer behaviour. You have also learnt about the importance of competitive analysis and the need for social marketing to look critically at the negative impacts of commercial marketing – especially in the hands of the hazard merchants. These are the two sides of the social marketing coin: borrowing ideas from commerce on the one hand, but critiquing and controlling it on the other. Both levers are then used to encourage beneficial health behaviour and, ultimately, social change.

References

Cannon T (1986) *Basic Marketing. Principles and Practice*. London: Holt, Rinehart & Winston.

Department of Health (2004) *Choosing Health: making healthy choices easier*. London: DoH.

Grönroos C (1994) From marketing mix to relationship marketing: towards a paradigm shift in marketing. *Management Decision*, 32 (2): 4–20.

Hastings GB, Elliot B (1993) Social marketing in practice in traffic safety, Chapter 3 in *Marketing of Traffic Safety*. Paris: OECD.

Hastings GB, MacFadyen L, Anderson S (2000) Whose behaviour is it anyway? *Social Marketing Quarterly*, VI(2): 46–58.

Jobber D (2001) *Principles and Practice of Marketing*, 3rd edn. Maidenhead: McGraw-Hill.

Kotler P, Zaltman G (1971) Social marketing: an approach to planned social change. *Journal of Marketing*, 35: 3–12.

Lazer W, Kelley E (1973) *Social Marketing: Perspectives and Viewpoints*. Homewood, IL: Richard D. Irwin Inc.

McDermott L *et al.* (2005) *A Systematic Review of the Effectiveness of Social Marketing Nutrition and Food Safety Interventions*. Stirling: Institute of Social Marketing, University of Stirling.

Morgan RM, Hunt SD (1994) The commitment-trust theory of relationship marketing. *Journal of Marketing*, 58: 20–38.

Richardson F (2001) Packages: the money or the options. *Business Review Weekly*, 23(20).

11 | Community development

Overview

This chapter describes how health promotion practitioners can adopt a community development approach to their work. Community development can be considered both a method and a philosophy for health promotion. It requires the health promoter to enable those whose health is at stake to participate in decisions about how to address their own health issues. Community development programmes seek to empower communities to develop solutions to the issues that affect them. This approach is particularly appropriate when addressing the health needs of socially disadvantaged communities. Community development programmes often seek to address the underlying structural factors that create the conditions leading to poor health. You will learn about how to plan and implement a community development approach to health promotion by reflecting on the experiences of programmes that have adopted these principles in rural South Africa.

Learning objectives

After reading this chapter, you will be better able to:

- explain the principles of community development programmes
- plan a health promotion programme based on community development principles
- describe the range of activities in which community development health promoters are engaged
- describe strategies to maximize the sustainability of community development approaches to health promotion
- describe the challenges and opportunities inherent in adopting a community development approach to health promotion

Key terms

Community A neighbourhood and/or group with common interests and identity.

Community development The process of change in neighbourhoods and communities. It aims to increase the extent and effectiveness of community action, community activity and agencies' relationships with communities.

Participation A process through which stakeholders influence and share control over development initiatives and the decisions and resources which affect them.

The principles of community development

> Rural development is the participation of people in a mutual learning experience involving themselves, their local resources, external change agents, and outside resources. People cannot be developed. They can only develop themselves by participating in activities which affect their wellbeing. People are not being developed when they are herded like animals into new ventures.
>
> (Nyerere 1968)

Families and communities have always made decisions regarding their health. In the twentieth century, responsibility for the health of communities has increasingly been placed in the hands of health professionals. A focus of health promotion has been the development of a more balanced situation where communities are empowered to promote their own health and support the interests of their most vulnerable members. This requires a radical change in attitudes to health. The community development approach to health promotion addresses the process of transformation in communities.

Putting community development into practice is based on a number of guiding principles. Core to these is the importance of benefiting the least empowered. Drawing on previous work in this area (Swannepoel 1997), these principles are:

- *The principle of human dignity*: community development programmes recognize that people have the ability to make their own decisions and take responsibility for their actions. Humans are seen as having many skills as well as needs.
- *The principle of participation*: community development programmes seek to make use of local knowledge, and maximize the sustainability of projects by ensuring people have a stake in their development. Yet facilitating participation is not easy: how can everyone participate, including groups such as the poorest of the poor? Participation can never be forced and all levels of participation are necessary in any project.
- *The principle of empowerment*: while using people's local knowledge in programme planning does not in itself promote empowerment, involving all members of a community in decision-making does. Participation without power is not the goal of development, but participation as an outcome of empowerment is. Community development programmes seek to equip people with the knowledge, skills and support necessary to allow them to participate in decisions at the level of their choice.
- *The principle of ownership*: while an external change agent (often a community health promoter) may facilitate identification of needs and the initiation of projects, achieving sustainability requires that ownership of these processes be transferred to the community itself.
- *The principle of learning*: community development programmes emphasize that all those engaged at all levels must learn from the process.
- *The principle of adaptiveness*: health issues and the context in which they develop change over time. Programme participants need to be willing to learn and adapt as they go forward. Mistakes should be seen as learning opportunities.
- *The principle of relevance*: community development programmes do not eschew new technologies yet they are not generally concerned with the discovery of these innovations. Rather, community development programmes recognize that technologies may require adaptation to and appropriate promotion in the

local context to maximize their relevance. Community development programmes facilitate local involvement in this adaptation and promotion process.

The decision on how to act within a given situation can be made upon reflection on
these principles. But adopting the principles of community development is not
always easy. While community health promoters must keep such principles in the
back of their mind at all times, not all principles are attainable at the same time and
it may be necessary to work on some before others are attained.

Delivering community development

Now you will see how the principles of community development are used in health
promotion programmes. You will learn how to *plan*, *work in* and *sustain* a community development health promotion programme. To facilitate this, you will
read about three health-related community development projects in rural South
Africa.

Following the first democratic elections in South Africa in 1994, community
development principles were entrenched in a number of policy documents in the
country, such as the Batho Pele ('People First') strategy for health services (Department of Public Service and Administration 1997). The projects you will learn about
were implemented in this generally supportive policy environment. Yet the
examples also show many of the complexities of adopting this way of working.
After reading about each of the case study projects you will be asked to reflect on
how a community development approach might also be applied to a new health
promotion programme targeting a health issue in your own field of interest.

Planning to use a community development approach

The Community Rehabilitation Research and Education Programme (CORRE) was
started in response to a growing awareness that people with disabilities living in
rural areas of South Africa were not receiving adequate rehabilitation services.
CORRE decided to adopt a community-based approach focused on 'rehabilitation,
equalization of opportunities and social inclusion of all children and adults with
disabilities', in order to 'ensure that people with disabilities are empowered to
maximise their physical and mental abilities, have access to regular services and
opportunities and become active, contributing members of their communities and
their societies' (ILO, UNESCO, WHO 1994). A community development approach
to rehabilitation thus recognized that disability is not merely an individual mental
or physical problem, but has social, cultural and political dimensions. The programme applied these principles when planning the recruitment of community
health workers, their training and their employment opportunities after the
training programme was completed.

The programme decided that the best means of addressing deficiencies in rural
rehabilitation services was to recruit and train community-based rehabilitation
workers (CRWs). The recruitment process emphasized principles of community
participation and empowerment. Posters were placed in villages advertising the
planned recruitment of CRWs. The rehabilitation team from the local hospital

went to each village and acted out a role-play that portrayed the role CRWs could serve and explained what qualifications individuals would need for inclusion in the training programme. Application materials were left in village clinics and collected by the rehabilitation team. Candidates were interviewed in the community by a panel of community leaders, people with disabilities and hospital human resource personnel. By emphasizing participation at this early stage, it was hoped that the CRW would be seen as belonging to, and therefore accountable to, the community. Through this process, community members were empowered to have a say in the delivery of rehabilitation services in their community, while CRWs were empowered to deliver these services.

Planning for implementation of the training programme also utilized community development principles. Maximizing the participation of stakeholders was crucial. All three therapy disciplines (physiotherapy, occupational therapy and speech therapy) and their professional boards were involved in the decision for the project to go ahead and the development of the curriculum. The profile of different disabilities identified in a needs assessment survey underpinned the issues to be addressed by the CRW training programme. During the training programme, professionals from all three therapies were involved in teaching, with people living with disabilities in the target communities playing a key role, both in the classroom and during practical periods.

In planning for life after the training, it was also essential to emphasize the principles of community development. In order to train CRWs to work in rural areas with minimal supervision, a two-year course was instituted, markedly different from one-year CRW training programmes implemented elsewhere in the world. The course was run on a block-release system and students frequently returned to their home villages on practical blocks. Thus, people with disabilities and their families were involved with the students' learning, and were at the same time being empowered themselves through students imparting knowledge to the community (Concha and Lorenzo 1993). Ultimately the aim was that students would take up employment in their own villages. A partnership was formed with the department of health in order to ensure that the students were employed once they were trained, and therapists were aware of their responsibilities in supervising CRWs. CRWs graduating from the programme thus had immediate employment, meaning that their new skills could straight away begin to benefit the communities from which they had come and which had themselves invested in the training.

✎ Activity 11.1

Imagine that you intend to implement a community development project in an area of health promotion with which you are familiar. Who would you want to participate in the planning of this programme? How would you ensure that all stakeholders participated fully? How else would you implement the principles of community development in planning your programme?

Feedback

You should have considered what the tasks were that each stakeholder would need to perform and thus decided who in the community would need to be involved. Remember that service providers should often also be regarded as members of the community. A collaborative effort would need to be planned with all the key people, who would together decide how to run an effective recruitment drive and programme, that was transparent and adhered to community development principles. It would be important to make sure that the planning group all understood and agreed to the community development principles used to underpin the programme.

Working in a community development team

Teamwork is inherent to community development. Yet community health promoters often face a tension in their work in both seeking to lead a programme but also to cede responsibility for the programme to others. Thus, while collaborative decision-making is essential to community development, these programmes require leaders, whose job it is to facilitate programme development and adaptation where necessary. As Figure 11.1 shows, in successful community development initiatives, decision-making power gradually transfers from these leaders or programme champions towards the community and those they appoint as their representatives.

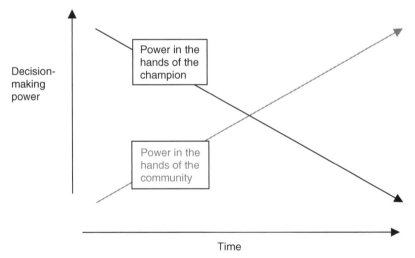

Figure 11.1 Transfer of decision-making power

A project was set up to improve the health of orphans and vulnerable children by increasing access to child grants which are available to poor families in South Africa. The project site was in a rural area of north-east South Africa, spread over about 300 square kilometers. Unemployment and poverty were common in the area and infrastructure was generally poor. Around a third of the population had been refugees from Mozambique and many lacked the vital documentation necessary to access child grants and other social support systems.

A two-year grant was obtained to evaluate a 'health camp' at which government officials would take applications for vital documentation and grants, health officers would assess the health of children and various service organizations would educate people about how to access their services. The community development worker was to implement this plan, facilitating the participation of local stakeholders and adapting the process to local needs.

To start the process, data made available by a local health research centre was presented to the heads of the relevant government departments. The data indicated that two of the major barriers preventing children from accessing grants were that service points for grant application were geographically inaccessible and that children lacked vital documentation (Twine *et al.* 2005). In order to address the first barrier, the head of the department of social security ensured that his department opened three social security offices in the project site where applications for grants could be made. Additionally, the social security officers based at these offices were invited by the community health worker to attend numerous community meetings to inform the community about grant application processes.

Over time, responses were increasingly adapted to local needs. It was suggested that the general population would not come to a single central health camp because of lack of transport and that resources would be better used in supporting relevant authorities to spend two days in each village with a team of volunteers taking applications for vital documentation and grants. This was organized, and the departments of home affairs and social security spent two days in each of 21 villages. Some 8000 people applied for documents during this campaign. Two small health camps were held and both community leaders and service providers appreciated these opportunities to share information and requested further such meetings.

Despite these successes, concern was expressed by a political councillor who had been observing progress that the scheme did not explicitly target orphans and vulnerable children. He called for a stakeholder meeting to discuss problems specific to these groups. A needs identification process conducted with the stakeholder group identified the following priorities: to identify why the application process for foster care and other grants took such a long time; to find ways to increase the numbers of people with relevant vital documents; and to investigate the misappropriation of food parcels that were meant for the poorest families. A task team was elected to look into these issues. Reporting on progress to the stakeholders biannually, the team collated information on services available to children, facilitated meetings between magistrates and social workers regarding foster care grants, and tried to collate information on food parcel provision held separately by the municipality and the local social workers. Ultimately, this task team oversaw the expansion of the home affairs outreach campaign to the rest of the district.

The project described above illustrates key principles of community development teamwork, such as participation and adaptiveness. Over time the project was increasingly directed by local government structures. The team increasingly developed a life of its own, and although the community development worker as a 'champion' remained the chair of meetings, tasks were undertaken by subcommittees without using donor funds. The programme also illustrates the process of transformation undergone by those involved in the project. Awareness was raised, leading to action, then reflection, then more action. As more people became involved, awareness of both the problems and the opportunities to deal with them grew.

 Activity 11.2

A remote community is identified as suffering a poor health profile in an area of health with which you are familiar. Imagine you are employed with a programme that wishes to use community development principles to address this issue. What would be your responsibilities? Who else would you work with? What challenges would you face? What information would you need and where might you access this?

 Feedback

The responsibilities you considered might have included finding out about current community leadership structures and what health and development services were currently available. You would need to interact with these structures and services and identify who could be part of a project team, and what roles they might play. A big challenge might be the level of community cohesion. You might seek to ensure representation of marginalized groups in existing structures. You would need to involve as many people as possible in all decision-making processes, and remember that people in the community already have much of the information you would require.

Sustaining community development programmes

Although community development principles are implicit in many important health promotion declarations some would argue that the hierarchical structure of large institutions such as departments of health prevents them from truly adopting these strategies. Consequently, a community development approach is most often adopted by relatively small organizations working in collaboration with communities. These organizations are often beset by many challenges. The sustainability of their efforts is often dependent upon continued support from external sources, such as funding agencies and health or development authorities, that rarely provide support to organizations for more than a few years at a time. Leaders of community development programmes thus need to consider strategies for sustaining the impact of their programmes. Community development practitioners can adopt a number of strategies to ensure their continued survival and maximize their impact. These strategies include fostering and nurturing *partnerships* with other organizations, conducting *evaluation*, monitoring and impact research, *responding to changes* in the context in which the programme operates and maximizing and diversifying *funding streams*.

In rural South Africa, a university-based HIV/AIDS control programme developed an HIV prevention programme. The programme sought to address factors in the socioeconomic environment that shaped vulnerability to HIV, specifically poverty and prevailing social norms on gender. A programme was developed with three component parts:

- a poverty-focused microfinance initiative for women in poor communities;
- structured training sessions on gender and HIV for microfinance clients;
- community mobilization activities developed with microfinance clients.

A strong partnership between the university HIV programme and the microfinance organization was essential in order to implement the project. A sense of ownership of the training component was promoted in the microfinance organization by conducting workshops with staff at all levels of the organization. A joint management committee was set up to provide a forum for problems to be raised and addressed. After a pilot phase of three years, the partners came together once again to plan a second phase of the work. Staff of both organizations were positive about the impacts the training programmes were having on microfinance clients, yet the sustainability of the programme was not assured. The university programme felt that long-term expansion of the programme was beyond its remit. In contrast, the microfinance organization was concerned about the financial and logistical impact of taking on responsibility for the training and its management. In response to these concerns, a second phase of work was planned in which increased responsibility for planning and managing the training component was taken on by the microfinance organization, while the university programme monitored aspects of this transfer to document lessons for all partners (Pronyk *et al.* 2005).

Evaluation and montoring exercises were used to maximize the impact of the programme and donors were provided with ongoing reports on progress. These efforts improved the likelihood that the programme would receive ongoing funding from existing donors. However, the longer-term sustainability of the approach required rigorous evaluation of whether the programme achieved its stated outcomes. Community development programmes are notoriously difficult to evaluate since they are highly flexible and have complex, often changing goals. Consequently many evaluations of these programmes have been small scale and/or qualitative. However, more rigorous attempts to document the outcomes of such programmes is necessary within a climate of evidence-based policy and practice. The first phase of this programme was conducted as a community randomized trial, the results of which were hoped to strengthen donor and government support for the approach (RADAR 2002).

After three years of programme activity, it became clear that the context of HIV vulnerability in the project area was changing. A large mining corporation had begun operations in the area. This shift in context created concerns. Mining has been associated with rapid HIV spread in South Africa and the project partners were concerned about the potential impact of these new developments on their HIV prevention work. However, the development also presented an opportunity to develop a partnership with the mining company, itself concerned with addressing HIV/AIDS issues in its work. After a series of consultations, funding was obtained to support an expansion of the programme in parallel with the development of mining activities. This increased the relevance of the programme to the project context, boosted and diversified its source of funding, and involved new stakeholders with an interest in the success of the programme.

Activity 11.3

Imagine you are responsible for maintaining the long-term survival of a community development programme addressing a health issue of your interest. Who and what could affect the sustainability of your efforts? What could you do to maximize your programme's sustainability?

Feedback

You might have thought that if community development principles are entrenched in the project then sustainability is being actively addressed. The more ownership community members and other stakeholders have in a project, the greater its chances of sustainability. However, community dynamics are constantly changing. You should have identified a number of stakeholders that could potentially affect your programme for good or for bad. Developing partnerships with these stakeholders and lobbying powerful bodies on issues of importance to your programme would be essential. Opportunities that arise out of other developments occurring within communities should not be overlooked. Having effective monitoring and evaluation structures would allow a greater ease of engaging with partners as dynamics change and projects take on a life of their own.

Strengths and weaknesses of community development

Community development is a relatively underused approach to health promotion. Yet a community development approach can lend strength to health promotion efforts in many situations where other approaches might be ineffective or impractical. Nevertheless, adopting a community development approach may not be appropriate in all situations. Such programmes face challenges in some contexts and a good practitioner needs to be aware of these potential weaknesses.

Strengths

Using a community development approach can:

- Ensure the effective uptake of new messages and technologies. Since there are often cultural and educational barriers to the introduction of new health messages or technologies, involving community members in their dissemination can maximize the chances that they are accepted.
- Have additional benefits for communities beyond the intended health benefits. In community development there is an emphasis on the process of generating a response to a health issue. By working with individuals to empower them to respond to a health issue, there are often additional benefits of value in their own right such as improved skills, knowledge or community involvement.

- Be sustainable. Successful community development programmes that ensure the participation of many stakeholders and facilitate community ownership of the solutions to health problems can be more sustainable in the long term.
- Promote health equity. Community development programmes often target the poorest communities, or the poorest people within communities. By reaching these groups, who are often left behind in other health promotion approaches, community development facilitates a more equitable distribution of health.

Challenges

Using a community development approach can:

- Be labour-intensive and difficult to implement on a large scale. Since community development programmes require local knowledge and need to be adaptable, these programmes are often coordinated through a single champion working in a relatively small area to ensure success.
- Be difficult to run. Stakeholders may not wish to participate in the process, health professionals may be unfamiliar with community development and project leaders may find it hard to let go of the programme. While such challenges are to some degree inevitable, early engagement with stakeholders affected by the goals of a new programme will help avoid problems later. Respecting local hierarchies such as chieftaincy or local government and seeking the support of leaders for the project at its inception is also a key step.
- Highlight conflicting priorities of community members. The expressed needs of different groups within a community may be in direct conflict with each other and with the remit of the community development worker. Dealing with such conflicting priorities is central to the continued success of community development initiatives. Community development workers must not give the impression that all needs can be addressed simultaneously. For this reason, it is often not a good idea to conduct needs assessments at big community meetings as this can produce unrealistic expectations and ultimately result in mistrust. Formative research and informal engagement with opinion leaders can help the community development worker identify and manage conflicting needs. Identifying clear aims for the project prior to community engagement, while not dictating processes, can help keep a project 'on target' in the early stages.
- Struggle to reach the most marginalized groups in a community. Reaching the most marginalized groups is a guiding principle for community development, but presents challenges. Marginalized groups may participate in community meetings, or their views may be deemed irrelevant. Community development workers must ensure the needs of such groups are documented and seek to learn from their ideas. As the process develops, community development workers might champion those needs and the skills that marginalized groups can bring to a project. Identifying complementary needs among all stakeholders may be an effective strategy for maximizing participation.
- Be difficult to evaluate. Community development programmes are complex and change according to community dynamics. Consequently it can be hard to identify what in a programme worked and what did not. There remains debate about the best way to evaluate such programmes. Nevertheless, monitoring and evaluation are central to any project plan. A streamlined monitoring plan

should document indicators of successful implementation in order to indicate the progress of the project to the implementers and beneficiaries, and identify areas for improvement. More rigorous evaluation strategies should be independently conducted since they will otherwise detract from the effective implementation of the programme.

• Take a long time to be effective. Community development initiatives often attempt to influence the underlying structural factors that affect health, and these may only change slowly. This can affect the motivation of all parties. Identifying realistic project aims as well as documenting successes along the way can help maintain energy.

 Activity 11.4

Imagine you are a community health worker in a rural village. Malnutrition is identified as a major source of children's ill health. Community members say that lack of employment is the main reason for this. Your supervisor suggests that working with teachers to train older children to maintain a vegetable garden might be a good entry point to deal with the problem. Yet six months later not a single vegetable has been harvested. While the children tell you they value the project, you are less certain that teachers are giving it their full support. What might have gone wrong? What could you have done differently? What should you do now?

 Feedback

You are faced with a difficult situation. Obviously you cannot generate higher levels of employment in an area, although the community has identified this as the underlying cause of the health problem. As such, you may indeed need to focus your efforts in one area. It would have been important to discuss what your project is able to contribute, both in public and privately with key opinion leaders. Reasons why teachers are not supporting the project may include: they are too busy; they are not getting support from their supervisors; they do not feel consulted; or the project may go against established community norms. Identifying such constraints early on would have been useful – but don't lose heart! Community development programmes need to adapt, and it would be important now to identify whether the programme can be improved or whether a different approach can be implemented within your project's remit.

Summary

You have read about three examples of a community development approach being used to address health problems, particularly in disadvantaged communities. Applying these principles in practice creates opportunities, but there are also significant challenges. Underlying all the programmes you have seen is the recognition that true development occurs only when people are involved in the process of development and activities that affect their lives and their health.

References

Concha ME, Lorenzo T (1993) The introduction of a training programme for community rehabilitation workers – the Wits/Tintswalo model. *The South African Journal of Occupational Therapy*, 23: 6–15.

Department of Public Service and Administration (1997) *Transforming Public Service Delivery White Paper (Batho Pele White Paper)*. Pretoria: Department of Public Service and Administration, Republic of South Africa.

ILO, UNESCO, WHO (1994) *Joint Position Paper on Community Based Rehabilitation*. Geneva: International Labour Organization, United Nations Education, Science and Culture Organization and World Health Organization.

Nyerere J (1968) *Freedom and Socialism*. Dar es Salaam: Oxford University Press.

Pronyk PM, Kim JC, Hargreaves JR, Makhubele MB, Morison LA, Watts C, Porter JDH (2005) Microfinance and HIV prevention: perspectives and emerging lessons from a community randomized trial in rural South Africa. *Small Enterprise Development*, 16: 26–38.

RADAR (2002) *Social Interventions for HIV/AIDS. Intervention with microfinance for AIDS and gender equity, evaluation monograph number 1*. Acornhoek: RADAR.

Swannepoel H (1997) *Community development: Putting plans into action*, 3rd edn. Kenwyn: Juta & Co. Ltd.

Twine R, Collinson MA, Polzer TJ, Kahn K (2005) Using the Agincourt Demographic Surveillance System in a rural South African district to measure equity of access to child support grants, a pro-poor government intervention. Working paper of the Agincourt Health and Population Unit, MRC/Wits Rural Public Health and Transitions Research Unit, University of the Witwatersrand, South Africa.

Overview

This chapter looks at the emergence of the settings approach, definitions, theory and practical steps to achieving health-promoting settings. These are addressed in the context of two well developed health-promoting settings: hospitals and schools, and with reference to workplaces, prisons and universities.

Learning objectives

After reading this chapter, you will be better able to:

- **explain the ways in which health promotion is put into practice in settings**
- **compare settings-based health promotion and intersectoral work**
- **describe different theories and ways in which settings-based work has been developed**

Key term

Settings for health The place or social context in which people engage in daily activities in which environmental, organizational and personal factors interact to affect health and well-being.

Introduction

The introduction of the terms 'health promotion setting', or 'settings-based health promotion' is usually attributed to the World Health Organization (WHO 1986). The theory and practice of healthy settings has been developed around the world and has been applied to interventions on defined groups or communities that include all the elements of the Ottawa Charter: action on policies, structural or system change within organizations, opportunities for increasing individual knowledge and skills and engagement with local communities.

Although the term is attributed to the Ottawa Charter phrase, 'Health is created and lived by people within the settings of their everyday life: where they learn, work, play and love', in fact it is actually initially stated in the section of the charter on 'Developing personal skills' – the theme referring to providing information, education for health and life skills: 'This has to be facilitated in school, home, work and community settings'. Much of the ensuing debate on the expansion of the concept of health education (which places responsibility on the individual to lead a healthy lifestyle) and health promotion (encompassing action on the social and environmental determinants of health and public policy), is played out in the ways in which health-promoting settings work. While the settings concept has enabled the operationalization of all of the Ottawa Charter's themes for health promotion, much discourse, and the reality of practice, falls short of the full realization of the potential of the concept to address action in all areas.

WHO further endorsed the concept in the Jakarta Declaration (WHO 1997) on *Leading Health Promotion into the 21st Century*. Here it was stated that: 'There is now clear evidence that . . . particular settings offer practical opportunities for the implementation of comprehensive strategies. These include mega-cities, islands, cities, municipalities, local communities, markets, schools, the workplace, and health care facilities'. Further: ' "Settings for health" represent the organisational base of the infrastructure required for health promotion. New health challenges mean that new and diverse networks need to be created to achieve intersectoral collaboration'.

So now 'settings' and 'sectors' are being used synonymously to describe different parts of society and their responsibilities to health. The differences and similarities between settings and sectors, and the relevance of the concept of health promoting settings will be explored in the exercise below.

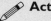 **Activity 12.1**

What do you think are the differences and similarities between promoting health in settings and through intersectoral collaboration?

 Feedback

There is general acceptance that both approaches move the focus from individual health problems and topic-based risk factors, to the system, or the organization. So as well as developing personal competencies, there is action on policies, partnership working and reshaping environments.

Grossman and Scala (1993) emphasize the organizational development processes and the importance of health promoters as change facilitators whose role includes 'organisational development, building intersectoral co-operation, negotiating and creating infrastructures'. However, Whitelaw *et al.* (2001) caution that there are significant differences in the breadth of work labelled as settings-based. They comment on:

> the sheer scale of the work (ranging from, for example, broad national approaches to highly localized work); the subsequent location of such work ('settings' ranging from, for example, nation states, cities, communities, schools, colleges, universities, health services/hospitals, workplaces and prisons) and, as is suggested by the diversity of the outcomes claimed in the name of settings

activity, the respective emphasis of each of the components of activity (ranging from broad policy and environmentally oriented work through to activity of a more individualistic and participative nature).

They suggest that the drive to develop settings-based models has created problems, including the grouping of widely differing activities together which may conceal differences in effectiveness and appropriateness for different contexts. The differences in scale and application may also make some practitioners feel their efforts fall short of the ideal.

Dooris (2004) queries whether the term 'settings for health' should be restricted to organizations, and if so, where do neighbourhoods, communities and cities fit in? Galea *et al.* (2000), describing work on healthy islands in the Western Pacific, also note concern about the growth of the concept until there is little in common between different types of setting. They suggest that:

A frame of reference for analysing settings must recognize that they exist in a hierarchy of different levels, with settings e.g. cities containing others e.g. schools. In such a frame of reference it is useful to consider an elemental setting as one which is indivisible for the purpose of organizing meaningful health promotion and health protection programmes. This elemental setting can be described as having three characteristics:

- it is small enough for its members to self-identify as belonging to that setting and to engender a sense of one identity;
- it has distinguishing social, cultural, economic and psychological peculiarities; and
- it has a recognizable, formal or informal administrative structure to which health promotion or health protection activities can link.

Elemental settings are contained within a broader contextual setting. Thus a city may contain important elements e.g. schools, hospitals and markets. Elemental settings directly affect the life of the people that live within them; they only affect others indirectly. An island is a contextual setting, itself enclosing other contexts (e.g. cities) and elements (e.g. schools).

They go onto assert that, 'Public health benefits accrue when effective action is taken both at the level of the elemental and contextual settings'.

Although the literature often includes healthy communities as settings-based initiatives, the definitions above more neatly capture the notion of a setting closer to an organization rather than a geographic area. While intersectoral working at municipality or city level is also essential, it is not the focus of this chapter. However, the recent WHO Bangkok Charter (WHO 2005), continues to use both terms, settings and sectors, without distinguishing them specifically.

Table 12.1 describes five types of settings-based health promotion, drawn from a review of activities in different settings (Whitelaw *et al.* 2001). These consider different perspectives of problems (the way in which the health 'concern' is perceived) and solutions, broadly whether the solution lies with the individual, or with the system or structure represented by the setting.

Table 12.1 Five types of settings-based health promotion

Type/model	Core perspective/ analysis of problem-solution	Relationship between the health promotion and the setting	Practical focus of activity
Passive	The problem and solution rest within the behaviour and action of individuals	Setting is passive: only provides access to participants and medium for intervention; health promotion occurs in setting independent of setting's features	Mass media and communication, individual education
Active	The problem lies within the behaviour of individuals, some of the solution lies in the setting	Setting provides 'active' and comprehensive resources to fulfil health promotion goals; health promotion utilizes setting resources	Mass media and communication, individual education plus complementary work on policy development and structural change around the specific topic area
Vehicle	The problem lies within the setting, the solution is learning from individually-based projects	Health promotion initiatives provide an appropriate means for highlighting the need for broader setting development; health promotion seen as a vehicle for setting change	Principle focus on developing policies and bringing about structural change using feeder activity from mass media and communication, individual education
Organic	The problem lies within the setting, the solution in the actions of individuals	Organic setting processes involving communication and participation are inherently linked to health and are thus 'health promoting'	Facilitating and strengthening collective/ community action
Comprehensive/ Structural	The problem and the solution lie in the setting	Broad setting structures and cultures inherently linked to health and are thus 'health promoting'; health promotion as central component of comprehensive setting development	Focus on developing policies and bringing about structural change

Source: Adapted from Whitelaw et al. (2001)

Activity 12.2

Look at the five different models shown in Table 12.1. For each one describe an example of a type of activity that might fit the model. You can draw examples from any setting that you are familiar with, or from different settings.

Feedback

Whitelaw *et al.* (2001) see the 'passive' model as one where problems and solutions rest within voluntary control of the individual, and the setting is simply a neutral communications channel offering access to defined population groups. An example would be health education within schools, where the school provides the opportunity to regularly reach cohorts of young people to teach them about keeping healthy.

The 'active' model is seen as a variation of this theme where aspects of the setting actively support the changes required in the target group. So health education about smoking in schools might be supported by smoking policies; hand-washing for nurses would include leaflets and action on the environment through improved washing facilities, introduction of policies and staff training. Thus part of the problem and solution is with the individual but changes to the setting contribute to achieving it.

The 'vehicle' model is exemplified by an understanding that the problem and solution lie within the setting but that the route to achieving change is through incremental steps on specific topics. Thus 'health promotion projects are used as a secondary vehicle towards the primary aim of wider development within the setting'. An example might be health-promoting hospital projects where action on topics is used to develop a wider understanding in the organization of the benefits of development towards being a health-promoting organization.

The 'organic' model places more emphasis on the role of individuals within the organization in changing the system in the longer term. This is based on the assumption that within an organizational setting the system processes are built up from the multitude of actions of individuals and groups within it. The solution therefore lies with developing individuals and changing processes embedded within the system. Actions here might include improving staff communications and more generic (i.e. not topic focused) staff training programmes. This approach has similarities with community development methods and continuous quality improvement approaches.

Finally the 'comprehensive' model also aims to make structural and process changes within the organization, but considers these are largely not within the control of individual staff to influence, as in the organic model. The solutions lie with attention to the levers of overarching settings' strategies and policies, and actions of senior management.

In reality much settings-based work combines these approaches, and indeed the distinction may be to do with the stage of development. Thus tangible health promotion projects may be a precursor to engaging staff involvement and senior management commitment to more significant organizational changes in systems and structures.

Health promoting hospitals

The fifth strategy of the Ottawa Charter is to 'reorient health services'. In the 1990s the WHO supported the development of the Health Promoting Hospitals (HPH) Network to support a growing number of hospitals that were beginning to attempt to put this into practice. Implementation of this strategy means paying attention to the other four strategies of: developing healthy public policy; creating environments that are supportive of health; involving the community; and developing personal skills of staff, patients, families and the wider community within the hospital setting. The HPH Network endorsed the fundamental principles of the *Vienna Recommendations on Health Promoting Hospitals* (WHO 1997).

 A HPH should:

1. promote human dignity, equity and solidarity, and professional ethics, acknowledging differences in the needs, values and cultures of different population groups
2. be oriented towards quality improvement, the well-being of patients, relatives and staff, protection of the environment and a realization of the potential to become learning organisations
3. focus on health with a holistic approach and not only on curative services
4. be centred on people providing health services in the best way possible to patients and their relatives, to facilitate the healing process and contribute to the empowerment of patients
5. use resources efficiently and cost-effectively, and allocate resources on the basis of contribution to health improvement
6. form as close links as possible with other levels of the healthcare system and the community.

Johnson and Baum (2001) note that in practice, 'there have been many different interpretations of the concept and many of these have not incorporated the range of strategies suggested by the Ottawa Charter. Some examples of health promoting hospital practice have simply relied on behaviour change strategies and little else'. They offer a typology of HPHs based on research in Australia that distinguishes organizational approaches. They observed that types of health promotion activity undertaken could be grouped into five categories:

* patients and their families; through health education and health counselling;
* staff; such as staff immunization, healthy eating in canteens, lunchtime walking groups;
* the organization as a whole; occupational health & safety, smoking policies and infection control;
* the physical environment; such as waste management programmes and energy reduction programmes;
* the community served by the hospital; collaborative health education projects with targeted groups, provision of health information through the internet and information centre.

They also noted that the degree of organizational commitment made by the hospitals had an impact on the extent and nature of activities. Combining these showed four distinct approaches to HPHs (shown in Table 12.2).

 Activity 12.3

Looking at Table 12.2, consider the examples of activity under the four approaches and note the extent to which they fulfil the five strategies of the Ottawa Charter and the Vienna Recommendations for HPH. What might be the benefits of the different types, and can you identify what the barriers to implementation might be?

Table 12.2 The four types of organizational approaches to HPHs

Type 1	Type 2	Type 3	Type 4
'Do a health promotion project'	'Delegate health promotion to a specific division, department or staff'	'Being a health promotion setting'	'Being a health promotion setting and improving the health of the community'
	Becomes the responsibility of a specified division, department or workers. It is not integrated into the whole of the organization	Hospital health promotion programme	Hospital health promotion programme
Ad hoc activities may be oriented to:	Activities may be oriented to:	Activities concentrate on the setting:	Activities encompass the setting and the community:
• patient and family • staff • organization • physical environment • community	• patient and family • staff • organization • physical environment • community	• patient and family • staff • organization • physical environment	• patient and family • staff • organization • physical environment • community Staff work collaboratively with others (intra- and inter-sectorally)

Source: (adapted from Johnson and Baum 2001)

 Feedback

While doing a health promotion project does not shift the strategic approach to health promotion in a hospital (as projects may be isolated and the core values of the organization not affected) it may have a role in the hospital evolving towards becoming more health-promoting. Such projects may catalyse further organizational development. Barriers would include the lack of skills and resources to undertake health promotion, and lack of managerial support for initiatives in the absence of organizational commitment. Sustainability would also be a significant barrier.

Delegating health promotion to the role of a specific division, department or staff, while improving resource allocation, is often seen to lead to lack of penetration of activity elsewhere in the hospital or to other staff. Health promotion is seen as 'their job', and therefore its integration into the whole organization and its impact is limited.

Being a health promotion setting is the most common role seen in those hospitals that are part of the WHO HPH Network. It usually involves organizational commitment, resource allocation and a planned programme of activity, usually directed at the hospital environment and its immediate target groups. It is often characterized by the need to 'get our own house in order' before reaching out into the community. To reach this stage requires the commitment of senior management and the adoption of health promotion as a core value within the organization, overcoming the difficulties of pressing budget demands and delivery goals.

In the final type the hospital has not only integrated health promotion into organizational processes, but recognizes its responsibility to the wider community it serves. Taking this upstream view of prevention, understanding the relationships between the hospital and community (e.g. through considering local employment practices and basic skills training), and developing intersectoral and other collaborative relationships, remain significant challenges for the hospital setting.

In order to stimulate self-assessment and incorporation of health promotion activities into the organizational culture, promoting patient and staff health, supporting healthy environments and cooperating with the community, the WHO produced *Standards for Health Promotion in Hospitals* (WHO 2004):

- Standard 1 – management policy. The organization has a written policy for health promotion. The policy is implemented as part of the overall organization quality improvement system, aiming at improving health outcomes. This policy is aimed at patients, relatives and staff.
- Standard 2 – patient assessment. The organization ensures that health professionals, in partnership with patients, systematically assess needs for health promotion activities.
- Standard 3 – patient information and intervention. The organization provides patients with information on the significant factors concerning their disease or health condition and health promotion interventions are established in all patient pathways.
- Standard 4 – promoting a healthy workplace. The management establishes conditions for the development of the hospital as a healthy workplace.
- Standard 5 – continuity and cooperation. The organization has a planned approach to collaboration with other health service levels and other institutions and sectors on an ongoing basis.

Using standards and a quality assessment process is valuable in the hospital setting as it parallels similar quality assurance approaches for clinical audit and service improvement.

✎ Activity 12.4

Do the WHO standards for health promotion in hospitals fulfil the overall aspirations of the HPH initiative and if not what more needs to be added? Do you consider them to be a practical starting point for hospitals to deliver comprehensive health promotion services, or are they over-ambitious?

Feedback

The WHO recognize that to address the complex interactions between hospital, community and environment will require further work, so these standards are focused on the main hospital health promotion activities, and hence are called standards for health promotion *in* hospitals. They do not cover issues of the wider impact of the hospital on the local environment and employment, or procurement of services and goods, in a health-enhancing and sustainable way. The community connections are primarily restricted to improved health promotion work within the hospital ensuring it is joined up with and draws upon community support and services for patient benefit. Given the limitations of some responses to HPHs and the dangers of marginalized 'projectism', the adoption of and adherence to these standards would be a great improvement in many hospital settings.

Health-promoting schools

As with hospitals, WHO has been instrumental in supporting global and regional networks to develop the health promoting schools concept. Based on the Ottawa Charter endorsement of the school as a setting for health promotion, and the development of whole-school approaches to health promotion, health promoting schools have become widely supported in many countries.

The whole-school approach recognizes that both the explicit (or formal) curriculum, and the hidden curriculum (what is learnt at school from norms, values and school life) are important in promoting health. The health-promoting school takes this a stage further to develop the 'hidden' curriculum into openly stated health-enhancing policy. For example, in England following the successful involvement of over 10,000 schools in the National Healthy School Standard, in 2004 the government announced that every school would become a healthy school. Progress had built on solid foundations of accredited local education and health partnerships, and joint working at national level between the education and health departments in government. A specific guide to healthy school status was issued in 2005 (www.wiredforhealth.gov.uk). Extracts are reproduced here as an example of a national government policy to support the development of health-promoting schools.

Note that as this is a national initiative it makes reference to UK government policies and mechanisms. For example 'Ofsted' is the national body responsible for assessing standards in education. Mechanisms may differ in other countries. Note which sectors of government or NGOs might help to support healthy schools where you are.

 1 National Healthy School status – a guide for schools

1 This guidance is for all schools

It outlines the National Healthy Schools Programme (NHSP), introduces the concept of national healthy school status and describes the benefits of becoming a 'healthy school'.

2 The aims of the National Healthy Schools Programme

- To support children and young people in developing healthy behaviours
- To help to raise pupil achievement
- To help to reduce health inequalities
- To help promote social inclusion

3 The benefits of being a 'healthy school'

3.1 A healthy school promotes the health and well-being of its pupils and staff through a well-planned, taught curriculum in a physical and emotional environment that promotes learning and healthy lifestyle choices.

3.2 Evidence of impact demonstrates that pupils who are healthy achieve well at school:

- schools can use the NHSP whole school approach to bring about sustained school improvement
- schools with healthy school status have better results for all Key Stage 1 assessments and Key Stage 2 Science compared with other schools
- schools involved in the NHSP are more inclusive
- pupils in healthy schools report a range of positive behaviours such as diminished fear of bullying and a reduced likelihood of using illegal drugs
- Personal, Social and Health Education (PSHE) provision is enhanced
- there is more effective liaison between home and school, and school and external support agencies

4 Healthy schools and reporting achievement

4.1 From September 2005, Ofsted will expect schools to demonstrate how they are contributing to the five national outcomes for children – being healthy; staying safe; enjoying and achieving; making a positive contribution; and economic well-being. Gaining national healthy school status provides rigorous evidence of this, and will assist you in evidencing your self-evaluation and completing your new school profile.

4.2 The NHSP builds on what schools have been doing for several years. The criteria referred to in this guidance complement existing and increasingly mainstreamed efforts to promote PSHE, physical activity, healthy eating and emotional health and well-being in the school setting.

5 Schools already involved with the National Healthy Schools Programme

5.1 Thousands of schools are already involved with their local healthy schools programme, and many have already been accredited by them. However, the government's intention is to introduce more rigorous and nationally consistent criteria through the introduction of national healthy school status. This guidance will enable schools to see how their current work is already contributing to the new healthy schools status.

6 Government commitment

The NHSP is funded by the Department for Education and Skills and the Department of Health, with a regional and local network. By 2009, the Government wants *every* school to be working towards achieving national healthy school status. The Government has ensured that every Local Education Authority already has a local healthy schools programme to support schools in reaching this target. From this year (2005) additional resources will be allocated to local programmes to support their work with schools. Each school will have access to a local healthy schools coordinator to support schools through the improvement process.

7 Links to other policies and programmes

Achieving national healthy school status enables your school to demonstrate its contribution to the five national outcomes for children and supports the targets within the following national priorities:

- improving behaviour and attendance
- improving performance in national Standard Attainment Tests
- reducing and halting the increase in childhood obesity
- promoting positive sexual health and reducing teenage pregnancy
- reducing young people's drug, alcohol and tobacco use

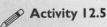 **Activity 12.5**

What elements that have been put in place to support schools (the goals of the programme, its adherence to the principles of settings-based health promotion and any other factors) are required for the success of the NHSP?

 Feedback

Some of the successful features you may have noticed include:

- cross-government policy and commitment
- national support *and* local programmes resourced to work with local schools
- focus on both priority health issues *and* educational achievement
- evidence of effectiveness
- history of development
- clear targets and criteria for achievement
- integration with national standards monitoring (Ofsted) recognizing the connections between health and educational standards
- actions on the curriculum e.g. PSHE, and on the environment
- a whole-school approach, and involvement of all staff, pupils and parents, and the wider community
- an organizational development approach of school improvement including review and action planning

How well, however, this type of 'top-down' approach compelling schools to be 'healthy' both adheres to the principles of settings-based health promotion and whether it will be successful in embedding it into everyday practice, is questionable.

Workplaces, universities and prisons

Health promoting workplaces have grown out of well established programmes to improve employee health, and now increasingly recognize their importance to wider considerations of sustainable social and economic development. Reviewing progress, Chu *et al.* (2000) note familiar distinctions between different types of activity:

- as a strategy of behaviour prevention in the workplace (lifestyle approach);
- as a part of extended occupational safety and health;
- as a strategy to influence important health determinants at work;
- as a strategy to reduce absenteeism;
- as a part of organizational development.

They identify success factors for workplace health promotion including: participation of all staff; project management including needs assessment, priority setting, monitoring and evaluation; integration into the organization's regular management practices; and comprehensively covering activities that are directed at both individuals and the environment.

Recently, health-promoting prisons and universities have begun to be developed. Both fit the definition of having defined boundaries and organizational structures and a clear population group. Health-promoting universities are important because of their scale in numbers of staff and throughput of students, and their impact on the local community. A strategy for health-promoting prisons in England aims to tackle the significant levels of physical and mental ill health in the prison population by paying attention to: mental health promotion and well-being; smoking; healthy eating and nutrition; healthy lifestyles including sex and relationships; and drug and other substance misuse. Working in partnership with the local health service this enables access to some of the most vulnerable and socially excluded in society.

The Health in Prisons Project (www.hipp-europe.org) is another WHO European network of similar initiatives. The WHO suggest that the successful mechanisms for sustainable health promotion in other settings will be effective in prisons. It recommends five key components:

- top management recognition and support;
- a multi-disciplinary group to assess needs, produce overall strategy and policies, plan and oversee implementation, measure success and revise policies;
- an implementation framework involving all staff, activities and regimes;
- opportunities to exchange ideas and experiences with others, to cooperate and to benefit from their experience, both within the prison service and outside;
- willingness to help develop standards.

The following example describes the approach taken in a prison in England. The role of Health Development Co-ordinator at Her Majesty's Prison Kirkham focuses on the strategy 'Health Promoting Prisons: a shared approach' and the associated Prison Service Order (PSO 3200), which advocate a 'whole prison approach' to health promotion – very much a settings model.

The priorities within this role were to ensure that health promotion became everyone's business, rather than purely a health care issue and to develop some multi-agency working in the field of health promotion in the prison setting.

An early mapping exercise of health promoting activity was useful in both identifying gaps and unmet needs and in illustrating the range of activity which can be considered to be health-promoting.

A multi-agency health promotion group has been meeting since August 2003 and a strategy and action plan has been developed and implemented with initiatives including a joint PCT/education healthy living course, smoking cessation, review of menus, new smoking policy, a commissioned health needs and assets survey and a health promotion fair.

Future plans include a prisoner-led health newsletter, peer health educators, a diversity week and the implementation of a mental health strategy. Promoting health in this context also means taking an active role in prison policy, strategy and working groups such as those for anti-bullying, self-harm, health and safety and diversity. This goes some way to ensuring that health, in its broadest sense, is integrated throughout the prison system and structures.

 Activity 12.6

Considering the examples of settings-based health promotion you have read, what concerns might there be about their implementation? Are they an effective mechanism to deliver both individual and organizational change? Are there population groups that might be missed out?

 Feedback

As the examples show, there is a danger that settings-based work is limited to a focus on individual behaviour change, conveniently delivered in a discrete organizational setting to a captive audience without having longer-term effects on the determinants of health. There is also concern that the organizational focus of the approach may exacerbate health inequalities. Children who truant or are excluded from school may miss out; equally the unemployed or those in small businesses may not be covered by such schemes.

As key features of success are similar across different settings they should be transferred to less accessible organizational settings. Also as individuals move between settings during their daily lives, health promoters should consider how to join up the learning from implementation of different settings programmes in localities.

Summary

You have learnt how the settings approach emerged, its definition, theory and practical steps to achieving health promoting settings with regard to well developed and evaluated health promotion settings. The differences and similarities between intersectoral and settings-based work have been considered, and different models of settings-based work discussed. You have seen that while health promotion projects within a setting may well be a useful step towards developing the setting to become health-promoting, they do not constitute what we think of as 'settings-based health promotion'. This needs to encompass organizational development having an impact on policies and practices within the organization, and on the wider community it serves. There are now recognized standards of practice for different settings, guidelines and extensive examples from different countries that all point to the transferability and value of this approach in delivering health promotion.

References

Chu C, Breucker G, Harris N *et al.* (2000) Health-promoting workplaces – international settings development. *Health Promotion International*, 15(2): 155–67.

Dooris M (2004) Joining up settings for health: a valuable investment for strategic partnerships? *Critical Public Health*, 14(1): 49–61.

Galea G, Powis B, Tamplin S (2000) Healthy islands in the Western Pacific – international settings development. *Health Promotion International*, 15(2): 169–78.

Grossman R, Scala K (1993) *Health Promotion and Orgnisational Development: Developing Settings for Health*. Copenhagen: WHO Regional Office for Europe.

Johnson A, Baum F (2001) Health promoting hospitals: a typology of different organisational approaches to health promotion. *Health Promotion International*, 16(3): 281–7.

Whitelaw S, Baxendale A, Bryce C *et al.* (2001) 'Settings' based health promotion: a review. *Health Promotion International*, 16(4): 339–53.

WHO Health Promoting Hospitals Network (1997) *The Vienna Recommendations on Health Promoting Hospitals*. Copenhagen: WHO Europe.

World Health Organization (1986) *The Ottawa Charter for Health Promotion*. Geneva: WHO.

World Health Organization (1997) *The Jakarta Declaration on Leading Health Promotion into the 21st Century*. Copenhagen: WHO.

World Health Organization (2004) *Standards for Health Promotion in Hospitals: Self-assessment Tool*. Copenhagen: WHO.

World Health Organization (2005) *The Bangkok Charter for Health Promotion in a Globalized World*. www.who.int/healthpromotion/conferences/6gchp/bangkok_charter.

13 Healthy public policy

Overview

Research has repeatedly demonstrated the importance of social conditions in influencing the health of individuals and populations. Government policies are major drivers of social conditions, and of public health and health inequalities. This chapter considers how government policies – such as housing, transport, income, education and welfare policies – may contribute to health, and gives examples of how they may reduce, and sometimes increase, health inequalities. It also considers the role of health impact assessment (HIA) in making policy healthier, and discusses how better evidence on healthy public policy can be obtained.

Learning objectives

After reading this chapter, you will be better able to:

- explain how policy may create the conditions for better, or worse, health
- describe some of the challenges to assembling evidence on healthy public policy
- give practical examples of how policy may be made more healthy

Key terms

Health inequalities Differences in health experience and health status between countries, regions and socioeconomic groups.

Social determinants of health Conditions which affect people's health such as their working and living environments, income, social networks and social position.

Social determinants of health

Public health policy in many countries is increasingly concerned with health inequalities. While population health is often improving, there are systematic differences between the most and least advantaged in terms of their health. The reasons for these health inequalities are widely accepted to lie predominantly 'upstream' rather than 'downstream'; that is, in the social determinants of health such as public policies, and people's social and economic circumstances rather than in individual risk factors, such as smoking or physical inactivity. The social determinants which are seen as most important vary from country to country (and from author to author) but some of the major determinants include:

- The social gradient: people further down the social ladder usually run at least twice the risk of serious illness and premature death as those near the top.
- Social exclusion: results from racism, discrimination, stigmatization, hostility and unemployment. These processes prevent people from participating in education or training, and gaining access to services and citizenship activities.
- Work: in general, having a job is better for health than having no job. But the social organization of work, management styles and social relationships in the workplace all matter for health.
- Unemployment: job security increases health, well-being and job satisfaction. Higher rates of unemployment cause more illness and premature death.
- Social support: social support helps give people the emotional and practical resources they need.
- Diet: social and economic conditions result in a social gradient in diet quality that contributes to health inequalities. People on low incomes, such as young families, elderly people and the unemployed, are least able to eat well.
- Transport: healthy transport means less driving and more walking and cycling, backed up by better public transport (adapted from Wilkinson and Marmot 2003).

 Activity 13.1

What social determinants – other than those mentioned above – are likely to affect health? Are there particular government policies (outside of the health sector) that you can think of in your own country that have the potential to improve health or to harm it?

 Feedback

The list of social determinants above is not exhaustive and there may be specific government policies which are likely to affect health. Policies influencing tobacco use – such as restrictions on smuggling and taxes – may be one example, though as we shall see below these may not work as expected. Some important social determinants have received little attention, such as peace and war, and there are international policies and agreements which have the potential to affect health, such as international trade agreements, which will also be discussed later.

Interest in the social determinants of health can be traced to the 1970s, when social researchers became increasingly critical of the narrow focus of public health research, which seemed to concentrate on disease processes and health care interventions, rather than on the role of the wider social and physical environment. In terms of advocating the potential of public policy as a tool for health promotion, Nancy Milio's book *Promoting Health through Public Policy* (1981) is often heralded as an important milestone and in 1986, using policy to promote health was taken up in the Ottawa Charter: 'Health promotion goes beyond health care. It puts health on the agenda of policy makers in all sectors and at all levels, directing them to be aware of the health consequences of their decisions and to accept their responsibilities for health' (WHO 1986).

Nearly 25 years later, in 2005, the Bangkok Charter emphasized again that health is the business of all sectors: 'Health determines socio-economic and political development. Therefore governments at all levels must tackle poor health and inequalities as a matter of urgency . . . Responsibility to address the determinants of health rests with the whole of government, and depends upon actions by many sectors as well as the health sector' (WHO 2005).

The idea that the health of the public can be affected, intentionally or otherwise, by the actions of planners or policy-makers is of course not unique to the twentieth century. Concern about social class gradients in health, and how these may be produced (and ameliorated), goes back centuries, at least to statistical investigations of the social patterning of mortality carried out in the seventeenth century. In 1842, Edwin Chadwick made clear the need for government to take responsibility for improving the living conditions of the poor in Victorian England. As well as documenting appalling living conditions, his report pointed to extensive inequalities in health between urban and rural dwellers. This helped create the conditions that led to the Public Health Act of 1848, which resulted in improvements in sanitation, sewerage and public administration. Chadwick's work emphasized the impact of poor living conditions on life expectancy, and drew on comparative international data, an approach still common among public health researchers today. He went on to detail the public savings that improvements in sanitation would produce. Like the Bangkok and Ottawa Charters, Chadwick's report recognized that the relationship between health and socioeconomic development is reciprocal: not only do social conditions promote health, but health is the bedrock on which social and economic development occurs. Chadwick's themes, of equity, the role of public policy and the potential cost-effectiveness of public health measures, have clear echoes in modern reports (e.g. Wanless 2004).

In the UK, the recent 'Programme for Action on Health Inequalities' (Department of Health 2003) gives some specific examples of how policy and cross-sectoral intervention can aim to reduce health inequalities. It points to examples of major cross-government programmes intended to target health inequalities, notably the Sure Start programme for children under 5 years living in disadvantaged areas, the Neighbourhood Renewal programmes and the UK Fuel Poverty Strategy. Before the Sure Start programme was rolled out, research evidence on the kinds of interventions which might make a difference was gathered. This was probably one of the most comprehensive attempts in the UK to use research evidence in rolling out a government programme.

The Programme for Action also emphasizes that health care organizations have an important role in improving public health and tackling health inequalities. The UK National Health Service (NHS), for example, has a key role to play in reducing inequalities in health resulting from injuries and illnesses where effective interventions can improve recovery and save lives. However, the general consensus for some decades has been that the greatest contribution to the health of the public is likely to come from developing *healthy public policy*, rather than from *health policies* and *health services* alone.

The unintended negative effects of public policies

One of the key concerns about public policy is the potential for unintended negative effects on health, and in particular the possibility that well-intentioned policies may unwittingly increase inequalities in health by having a greater impact on the better off. Health education is one often-cited example; it is argued that the generally better educated middle-classes are likely to benefit more from the provision of health information to a population and so provision of information in this way may actually risk increasing health inequalities (Wanless 2004).

Policies to control smoking are another example. Tobacco control policies in the UK since the 1970s have been accompanied by widening gaps between manual and non-manual socioeconomic groups. It is therefore essential that interventions to prevent the uptake of smoking, or to promote smoking cessation, are effective among disadvantaged groups, and do not contribute to a continuing widening of inequalities. Current approaches to reducing smoking tend to concentrate on the target of reducing overall tobacco consumption, rather than addressing the persistently large gap between smoking rates in higher and lower socioeconomic groups.

Taxes on cigarettes are often seen as an important means of controlling smoking, but a government commissioned report on public health in the UK (Wanless 2004) has examined how taxes and subsidies might be used by government more generally as levers to improve health. One example given by Wanless is the taxation of potentially unhealthy foods. Increasing the tax on foods with high levels of salt and fat might be used in an attempt to reduce their consumption. However he warned that whether or not such benefits would materialize in practice depends on two factors. First, there is not usually a simple relationship between one type of food and health outcomes, so it is not clear that simply taxing fatty foods would lower obesity or reduce rates of coronary disease. Second, consumers and producers would find ways to avoid new taxes in ways that do not necessarily promote healthier behaviour. We know in the case of cigarettes that taxation often results in tobacco smuggling, so cheap cigarettes remain available. As an alternative to taxes, subsidies can be used to promote health behaviours but these too can contribute to the creation of inequalities as an example from the Wanless Report (2004) illustrates:

Given the positive externalities associated with physical exercise, it could be argued that gyms should be subsidised. Though there is a case for government intervention to support physical activity, a simple gym subsidy is likely to be ineffective and inequitable because:

- subsidising gym fees, which are typically charged on a monthly basis and are not related to the amount of exercise undertaken, could encourage gym membership without actually encouraging exercise;
- much of the subsidy would go to people who are already going to a gym or are likely to do so – the people who tend to be healthier; and
- gym membership is more prevalent in the more healthy middle-classes, and gyms are not found in all locations, so the subsidy will tend to assist certain healthier sections of society more, increasing health inequalities.

Inequalities are also a concern of the UK White Paper *Choosing Health: Making*

Healthy Choices Easier (Department of Health 2004). This White Paper looks forward to a society 'where more people, particularly those in disadvantaged groups or areas, are encouraged and enabled to make healthier choices', and describes how the government will have discussions with the food industry to ensure clearer labelling of packaged food, along with increasing provision of information on diet and nutrition. However, this move toward promoting choice has been seen by some as a retrograde step; after all, as described above, health education messages promoting individual choice may be taken up more readily by those who are well off, and well educated. From this perspective, a potentially healthy public policy – promoting individual choice through providing more and better information – may actually fail to support the most vulnerable groups in society. *Choosing Health* does however include examples of healthy public policies which support the development of healthy environments and thus may be protective of public health. For example, it commits the government to a comprehensive and effective strategy for action to restrict the advertising and promotion to children of foods and drinks that are high in fat, salt and sugar.

These examples illustrate several of the characteristics of healthy public policies: they should contribute to the creation of environments which are protective of the health of individuals and communities but they should not inadvertently cause harm to the public's health nor should they contribute to the creation or exacerbation of existing health inequalities. The need to identify whether policies are likely to be healthy or unhealthy, and to help policy-makers avoid some of the above pitfalls, led to the development of the field of health impact assessment, which is discussed below.

The role of health impact assessment

Health impact assessment (HIA) is an approach which aims to help with the identification of policies or other social interventions that have the potential to harm population health. HIA developed from a concern that major public policies could have negative health effects. The importance of HIA has been emphasized in successive World Health Organization (WHO) and European Union (EU) policy documents and in the UK has been advocated as a key means of addressing health inequalities. Although the range of activities described as HIA is broad, it is now taken to describe 'the prospective estimation of potential impacts of a proposed policy or programme on a population's health, or any combination of procedures or methods by which a proposed policy or programme may be judged as to the effects it may have on the health of a population' (Kemm and Parry 2004).

Broadly, HIA involves two key stages:

* *Screening*, in which policies, programmes or projects are assessed to determine whether they may have a health impact, and what type of impact. This may be done on the basis of expert knowledge and available evidence (Kemm and Parry 2004).
* *Scoping*, in which further information is sought on the potential direct and indirect health effects of the proposed policy, and in which the methods, resources, participants and the timeframe for the further HIA process are assessed.

These stages will then reveal the need for further work – for example, a *rapid health impact appraisal*, which is a systematic assessment of the health impact of a policy, programme or project by a number of experts, decision-makers and representatives of those potentially affected by the proposed policy. Alternatively, a *health impact analysis* may also be carried out, which is an in-depth examination of a policy, programme or project, its potential impact on health and of the opportunities for adjusting the policy, programme or project to ensure a more positive impact on health. Finally, where an in-depth analysis is not possible, a *health impact review* may be carried out, which aims to estimate the most significant health impacts on health of the policy, without attempting a detailed investigation of specific individual impacts on sub-groups. This may be based on a review of earlier published analyses of similar policies (where they exist), along with consultations with experts.

HIA has grown rapidly as a possible means for assessing the impact of policies on health inequalities and making public policy healthier. Numerous HIAs have now been published, and methods are subject to constant revision (e.g. Kemm and Parry 2004). However, whether HIA really succeeds in achieving healthy public policy in practice may be difficult to determine. Greater emphasis needs to be placed on the use of robust qualitative and quantitative approaches in HIA – including epidemiological techniques.

It is worth noting here that national policies are not the only driver of health inequalities. Labonte (2001) for example has described how inter-national agreements to promote free trade between countries can contribute to inequalities:

> There is little doubt the World Trade Organisation (WTO), and its growing number of trade, investment and 'trade-related' agreements, further circum-scribes the abilities of governments to pursue health and social development goals via economic policy variables . . . Both the EU and the US have threatened to use the WTO TBT (Technical Barriers to Trade) Agreement to prevent Japan from implementing legislation on automobile emissions as part of its Kyoto commitments . . . Part of the problem is that liberalisation is unequally practised. Wealthy nations remain protectionist in areas where it benefits their interests while demanding open markets where it harms only poorer nations.

✎ Activity 13.2

The EU Common Agricultural Policy (CAP) is often cited as an example of how European food policy can affect public health. The CAP was established to deal with food shortages after the Second World War by promoting intensive farming, support-ing rural economies and maintaining standards of living for rural communities (e.g. by maintaining prices for fruit and vegetables and protecting farmers from competition by taxing imports). How might measures such as these affect diet, health and health inequalities?

Feedback

Maintaining high prices for fruit and vegetables penalizes low-income consumers, and so could be regarded as an obstacle to equity. Also there are negative impacts on health of tobacco subsidies. One result of this over-production has been the export of low quality, high-tar tobacco (at the EU's expense) to less affluent countries, including many of the EU's neighbours in central and eastern Europe, which is both unethical and inequitable.

Evidence-based public policy

In the UK, the growth in HIA came during a period of great interest in evidence-based public policy (EBPP). At the core of EBPP is a demand that public policies should be developed, refined and implemented on the basis of sound scientific research. This emphasis on the importance of 'hard evidence' reflects a growing consensus that social policies and interventions should be based on robust evidence of 'what works', rather than on past practice, or received wisdom. Much public health decision-making and health promotion practice is based on plausibility, politics and timeliness, rather than on research.

There is a need to systematically review the evidence base about wider determinants of health and health inequalities, including government policies (e.g. Wanless 2004). There are, however, undoubted barriers to the instrumental use of evidence to support policy-making in this fashion. One is that the availability of robust evidence of effectiveness in many areas of public policy is often low. Quite often evidence on 'what works' is simply missing, most particularly evidence on health inequalities. Policy-makers themselves have pointed out that much of the current evidence on health inequalities available to them simply does not answer policy-relevant questions, in particular with respect to 'upstream' interventions relating to the broader social determinants of health (e.g. education, income, employment policies) (Petticrew *et al.* 2004). The most obvious gaps are those caused by the relative lack of evaluations of the effectiveness and cost-effectiveness of policy and other interventions.

 Activity 13.3

What other types of research evidence are needed to support healthy public policy-making?

 Feedback

Much of the evidence that is available to us is descriptive, such as observational studies. These describe the extent of health problems in the population and indicate where action is needed. Policy-makers themselves have pointed to the lack of quantitative outcome evaluations. However, this is not the only sort of research they perceive to be necessary; they also point to the need for predictive research (e.g. the development of predictive models exploring the costs and benefits of different policy options), for methodological research on the means of assessing the impact on health of clusters of interventions ('policy clustering') and for better qualitative evidence of the impacts of policies (Petticrew *et al.* 2004).

These criticisms provide some practical pointers for those interested in helping policy-makers develop healthy public policy. The first is that, in the absence of evaluative evidence, a wider evidence base needs to be drawn upon. Healthy public policy requires the integration of evidence from evaluations of interventions (where possible), but also descriptive epidemiological evidence – describing the relationship between determinants of health and health outcomes – and this needs to be informed by theoretical frameworks, describing plausible causal pathways between policies and their outcomes.

In policy circles different types of experimental and non-experimental evidence are often brought to bear on policy questions, and so it has been suggested that a priority for researchers should be to help policy-makers with managing this 'mixed economy' of evidence. The challenge of course is that a decision is not based on evidence alone; research provides only one source of support for policy. Nutley *et al.* (2002) warn that:

> simple and unproblematic models of EBPP – where evidence is created by research experts and drawn on as necessary by policy makers and practitioners – fail as either accurate descriptions or effective prescriptions. The relationships between research, knowledge, policy and practice are always likely to remain loose, shifting and contingent.

Moreover, not all policy decisions may require the same level of scrutiny of the evidence; minor policy decisions may be handled incrementally (sometimes referred to as 'muddling through') where only minor changes to policy take place, while the more consequential decisions are handled through 'mixed scanning', where a range of policy options are scanned and then further work to acquire and analyse relevant information takes place, focusing only on the more consequential policy options.

Nutley *et al.* (2002) suggest that the rational introduction of research evidence into the policy-making process is rare; modern policy-making is more often represented by interactive, enlightenment, political and tactical models of evidence use. They suggest six models of research utilization:

- *the knowledge-driven model*: research generates knowledge that impels action;
- *the problem-solving (or engineering) model*: involves the direct application of the results of a specific study to a pending decision;
- *the interactive/ social interaction model*: utilization occurs as a result of a complex set of interactions between researchers and users which ensures that they are exposed to each other's worlds and needs;
- *the enlightenment (or percolation) model*: research is more likely to be used through the gradual 'sedimentation' of insight, theories, concepts and perspectives;
- *the political model*: research findings are ammunition in an adversarial system of policy-making;

- *the tactical model*: research is used when there is pressure for action to be taken on an issue, and policy-makers respond by announcing that they have commissioned a research study on the matter.

Implicit in most of the models is the assumption that research-based evidence will actually be available; that is, it will exist in a recognizable, digestible and meaningful form, and that it can be located and brought to bear on decisions about how to tackle major public health challenges (such as health inequalities). This task is often far from straightforward however, and the challenges in collecting and synthesizing evidence to support healthy public policy can be illustrated by an example from the field of transport.

Healthy transport policy

Transport may have a major impact on population health and on health inequalities. Although there is a general emphasis within public health research on negative impacts associated with motorized road vehicles, wider public health impacts may be anticipated. These include community severance, such as reduced access to local amenities and disruption of social networks caused by a major road running through the community, along with social inequalities and increased disturbance among residents. Transport, however, is an essential part of people's lives, granting access and convenience that may improve well-being. This may help explain why, despite the harmful effects associated with automobiles, car ownership has been suggested in some cases to be beneficial to the owner's health. Meanwhile, physically active forms of transport, such as walking and cycling, are widely assumed to promote fitness and health, but less evidence is available on how a greater reliance on physically active transportation might affect people's risk of personal injury or their access to amenities. As transport issues, particularly road transport, often invoke strongly polarized views among health researchers, systematic reviews are valuable in providing a more objective method of research synthesis that aims to limit the effects of personal bias.

One systematic review has considered this issue (Egan *et al.* 2003). This review was based on 32 primary studies and included any study that attempted to evaluate the health impacts of opening one or more new roads on a population in a developed country. The population could be vehicle users, pedestrians and/or residents, and the health measures could include specific physical or mental health outcomes, or more general measures of personal well-being, such as satisfaction with the area or disturbance. The review found that new urban arterial roads tended not to affect significantly the incidence of accidents involving injury, although the adding of a new lane to an existing arterial road, along with intersection improvements, did reduce injuries. New urban arterial roads increased noise disturbance and community severance in local communities. Findings from a qualitative study suggested that residents may attempt to adapt to the increased disturbance by changing aspects of their behaviour, their home environment or their attitude to the increased traffic. However, the quantitative studies suggested that such forms of adaptation tended to have relatively little impact on residents' subjective experience of disturbance, and that disturbance could still be detected among residents at least three years after the opening of a new road. Opening out-of-town bypasses and other major roads and motorways going through rural areas reduced the incidence of injury accidents on main routes in those areas. Bypasses reduced disturbance among residents of bypassed towns, especially small towns, but there was some evidence that outside such towns, people living near the route of a new bypass experienced adverse effects.

Considering the evidence in this way can provide an objective assessment of the positive and negative impacts of public policies on health, but, in this review, evidence with respect to the effects of new road building on health inequalities was lacking. This is a common finding and is perhaps the greatest challenge to the production of evidence to tackle health inequalities. Jackson and Waters (2004) have indicated that systematic reviews have generally adopted a utilitarian focus: trying to identify interventions that will achieve the greatest health gains for the greatest number of patients or populations. Primary research is subject to a similar 'utilitarian bias'; for example, primary studies of the effects of tobacco control interventions (such as public policies) tend not to analyse the effects of those interventions by markers of social position (Ogilvie and Petticrew 2004). This may be due to a lack of understanding of the difference between the determinants of health and the determinants of inequalities in health, and how they may be created and reduced.

 Activity 13.4

Advocating healthy public policy is easy, but specifying exactly how specific policies can be made healthier is difficult. Given what we know about the social determinants of health, what policy measures might be taken to improve health?

 Feedback

Health may be improved through housing, neighbourhood renewal, environmental and education benefits, and transport policies. Earlier examples given in this chapter point to public policies on smoking control as having the potential for both positive and negative effects, and the use of HIA has also been advocated as one possible route for accentuating the positive effects and mitigating the negative effects of policies.

As for knowing whether these measures have the desired effects, finding evidence of the effectiveness of policies in improving health and reducing inequalities is usually challenging, as there are still relatively few evaluations of the outcomes of policies, and so decisions about the ways in which policies can be changed to improve health may often be based on theoretical frameworks describing the determinants of health, descriptive evidence and considerations of social justice, as much as on evidence of 'what works'.

Summary

This chapter has outlined some of the ways in which public health can be improved through policies and other influences from outside the health sector. It has also considered some of the barriers to healthy public policy – not least that in some cases international agreements and policies may have an important influence on public health. Evidence-based policy-making was introduced as a way of gathering better evidence on the health effects of policies, though it was acknowledged that the linkage between evidence and policy can be complicated. For researchers seeking to introduce better evidence of the health effects of public policies into policy development, the development of networks and cultivation of relationships between public health practitioners, advocates and policy-makers is a means of providing durable opportunities to influence the policy process.

Achieving healthy public policy clearly requires better evidence of the effects – positive and negative – of non-health sector policies, and of their distributional effects, but it also requires closer relationships between research and policy than is sometimes the norm and than both communities are sometimes comfortable with.

References

Department of Health (2003) *Tackling Health Inequalities: A Programme for Action*. London: Department of Health.

Department of Health (2004) *Choosing Health – Making Healthy Choices Easier*. London: Department of Health.

Egan M, Petticrew M, Ogilvie D, Hamilton V (2003) Health impacts of new roads: a systematic review. *American Journal of Public Health*, 93: 1463–71.

Jackson N, Waters E (2004) The challenges of systematically reviewing public health interventions. *Journal of Public Health*, 26(3): 303–7.

Kemm J, Parry J (2004) What is HIA? Health impact assessment, in J Kemm, J Parry, S Palmer, *Health Impact Assessment*. Oxford: Oxford University Press.

Labonte R (2001) Liberalisation, health and the World Trade Organisation. *Journal of Epidemiology and Community Health*, 55: 620–1.

Milio N (1981) *Promoting Health through Public Policy*. Philadelphia, PA: Davis.

Nutley S, Davies H, Walter I (2002) *Evidence Based Policy and Practice: Cross Sector Lessons From the UK*, ESRC UK Centre for Evidence Based Policy and Practice: Working Paper 9 (available at http://evidencenetwork.org/documents/wp9b.pdf).

Ogilvie D, Petticrew M (2004) Smoking policies and health inequalities. *Tobacco Control*, 13: 129–31.

Petticrew M, Whitehead M, Macintyre S, Graham H, Egan M (2004) Evidence for public health policy on inequalities: the reality according to policymakers. *Journal of Epidemiology & Community Health*, 58(10): 811–16.

Wanless D. (2004) *Securing Good Health for the Whole Population: Final Report*. London: HM Treasury (available at www.hm-treasury.gov.uk/consultations_and_legislation/wanless/consult_wanless04_final.cfm).

WHO (1986) *Ottawa Charter for Health Promotion*. Geneva: WHO (available at www.who.int/hpr/NPH/docs/ottawa_charter_hp.pdf).

WHO (2005) *Bangkok Charter for Health Promotion*. Geneva: WHO (available at www.who.int/healthpromotion/conferences/6gchp/hpr_050829_%20BCHP.pdf).

Wilkinson R, Marmot M (2003) Social determinants of health: the solid facts, 2nd edn. Geneva: WHO (available at www.who.dk/document/e81384.pdf).

SECTION 3

Delivery and reflection

14 Project planning and budgeting

Overview

Successful delivery of health promotion requires sound project management from planning through implementation to completion. In this chapter you will explore the different tasks involved in project management and how to undertake these tasks. In doing so, you will also learn about the importance of proper budgeting and budget monitoring and how to go about this.

Learning objectives

After reading this chapter, you will be better able to:

- **describe the key tasks involved in effective project management**
- **use different tools to facilitate project management**
- **develop SMART objectives**
- **prepare a project budget and monitor this**

Key terms

Plan A time-limited document describing programmes, strategies and projects and how they relate to each other.

Strategy A plan informed by evidence, values and theories that sets global and specific aims and describes how these will be achieved.

Why is project management important for health promotion projects?

A project management approach tends to be most closely associated with industry but it is particularly relevant to health promotion programmes and interventions for a number of reasons.

First, as discussed in Chapter 1, effective health promotion requires a multi-levelled or programmatic approach. This means that a health promotion programme will involve the interaction and interdependence of several projects. Unless each of these projects is well managed, the success of the other projects and the programme as a whole will be jeopardized.

Second, health promotion requires the involvement of many different participants and stakeholders. On a practical level, the success of the project will require input from individuals and agencies with relevant expertise and experience at the planning stage and throughout implementation. On an ethical level, potential users and beneficiaries of a project should be involved in decision-making. For this involvement to be meaningful it needs to be planned and managed to ensure the right people and agencies are involved at the right time.

Third, health promotion involves the investment of substantial sums of public money and remains an often controversial area. Health promotion agencies must ensure that this funding is used for the purposes for which it was allocated, that value for money is obtained and that money is properly accounted for. This requires proper budgeting and budget monitoring.

Fourth, health promotion involves an ethical imperative to be explicit about the rationale for an intervention and the assumptions, values and principles on which it is based (Speller 1998). This imperative can only be met if there is a clear and transparent process for developing and implementing projects.

Finally, the increased emphasis on evidence-based practice within health promotion means that it is important to show if the project successfully met its aims and objectives. This means the aims and objectives of a project need to be defined from the start.

A practical guide to project management

There are many different theoretical and technical approaches to project planning and management. These include logical frameworks, the precede-proceed model, the public health decision-making model (PABCAR) and the community organization model (Tones and Green 2004).

This chapter does not seek to explain these approaches in detail. Rather it offers a practical guide to project management that incorporates the main features shared by many of these project management models. In doing so it breaks the process of project management into three main stages:

- planning the project;
- implementing the project;
- completing the project.

Each of these stages is further broken down into a series of tasks. These tasks are described here in the order in which they usually follow on from each other, but several of them will need to be carried out simultaneously. Indeed some of the tasks will continue throughout the process of managing the project. Others will need to be revisited depending on the project's progress. In addition, the process of project management will need to be adapted to each project and will depend on different factors, including the size and complexity of the project, the capacity of the implementing agencies, the amount of funding, the number of different stakeholders and the impetus for developing the project. This means there is no 'one size fits all' model for project management.

Planning the project

Task 1: identifying the need that the project will address

The first stage is usually to identify the 'need' that the project seeks to address. In Chapter 2 you learnt about the different types of need (normative, comparative, felt and expressed) and the different methods for undertaking needs assessment. Before you can proceed to formulate the project's aims and objectives, you need to be clear about what needs the project seeks to address.

When you have identified the need you can go on to review evidence on how previous interventions have been used to meet similar needs. As discussed in Chapter 3, different methods may be effective in different settings and with different groups. In short, it is not possible to say some methods are 'effective' and others 'ineffective'.

Identifying need also involves an ethical dimension. Health promotion practitioners may experience a dilemma or tension between autonomy (the right to individual self-determination) and justice (fairness and equity). Inevitably there will be some situations where the former will need to be compromised for the latter. A classic example would be anti-smoking programmes which limit the right of individuals to smoke in certain places to protect the health of others. It is also important to avoid ideological or value-laden judgements about health need. A health promotion should not seek to influence behaviour because it is perceived as 'bad', but because of its negative impact on health. The best way to avoid such judgements is to be explicit about the need identified, whose need it is and why it is considered to require intervention.

Task 2: stakeholder analysis and engagement

Individuals and agencies that have an interest in a project are often called stakeholders. Stakeholders can be divided into three types (Tones and Green 2004):

- primary stakeholders: potential beneficiaries of the project;
- secondary stakeholders: those who may be involved in the project's delivery;
- key stakeholders: without whom the project cannot go ahead.

Ethically, it is essential that you engage with people who may be affected by the project at an early stage in development. Potential beneficiaries should ideally be involved in both designing *and* implementing a project which aspires to meet their needs.

After identifying agencies, groups and individuals who are potential stakeholders, the next step is to consider what they can potentially contribute to the project and how they can be actively engaged. The way you do this will depend on who they are and the nature of their interest in the project. Forms of stakeholder involvement include planning workshops, user-participation events and partnership forums. Stakeholders will need accessible information and facilitation for their participation to be meaningful. This should include information on the evidence base. Engagement with stakeholders takes time and needs to continue throughout the duration of the project.

Activity 14.1

Imagine you are involved in a project to improve the sexual health of teenage girls. Think about who the stakeholders may be and divide these into primary, secondary and key stakeholders.

Feedback

You should have included beneficiaries and organizations currently working with these beneficiaries, statutory agencies and funders. You should also consider whether there are agencies or individuals that might oppose the project.

Task 3: building a project team

Increasingly, projects are delivered by partnerships made up of organizations from different sectors. Organizations and sectors have different ways of working and individuals have priorities and commitments to their own organizations. Therefore, it is important to build commitment to, and a shared understanding of, the project among those involved. One way of doing this is to develop a project team made up of the key individuals from the stakeholder organizations. The project team should ideally work together to plan the project and individual members of the team may be responsible for implementing specific components of the project.

Complex or large projects may also require a project management or steering group. These will usually include the senior managers of the organizations involved in the project and can also include representatives of other stakeholders, such as beneficiaries. The role of a project management or steering group is to oversee the project's progress, provide accountability and bring senior commitment. Generally, the group meets regularly throughout a project's implementation. It approves the project plan and budget and any subsequent amendments. Although establishing such a group may seem like introducing an unnecessary layer of bureaucracy, it can be a useful way of avoiding conflict where there are complex interactions of agencies.

In many cases, a project comes from an idea at a multi-agency meeting. It may be discussed in several forums and different organizations may sponsor research into needs, a feasibility study and participation events. But before project implementation can commence, a decision should be taken as to who is the lead agency. This does not imply the lead agency must find all the required resources or take all the responsibility. However, to ensure good coordination, one agency must take responsibility for project management.

When the lead agency has been established, an individual from that agency should be assigned the role of project manager. The role of the project manager is crucial to the success of a project. This person coordinates the project, collates and disseminates information on progress, brings together the project team and/or project management or steering group. The work involved in being the project manager is commensurate with the size and complexity of the project but it is essential that the project manager has sufficient time and resources to carry out the role. For this reason, the function and responsibility should be included in that individual's formal work plan.

Developing a project team also requires capacity-building. Capacity-building is action to ensure the necessary resources, expertise and commitment exist for the project's successful implementation. It may include training for members of the project team and staff in partner organizations on the skills needed to implement the part of the project they are involved in. It could also involve team-building for the project management or steering group to build understanding of and commitment to the project. Capacity-building is also essential for the sustainability of the project.

If you need additional skills or capacity to implement the project, you may need to recruit new employees. When recruiting new employees it is important to be clear about what the overall role of the new staff member(s) will be and how this relates to the project's aims, what specific tasks they will be required to undertake and how they will be managed and supported. This should be laid out in a job description. You also need to develop a person specification that describes the skills, qualifications and experience the new staff member(s) will need to have to carry out the job successfully. To get the right person for the job, it is essential you develop a job description and person specification before you begin recruitment. Recruitment should be undertaken in such a way that all potential candidates are given equal opportunities.

Task 4: defining the aims and objectives

Overall health promotion aims are usually broad and achievable only by an overall programme rather than by one project alone. For example, the overall aim of a healthy eating programme might be to bring about reductions in childhood obesity. The aim for a project making up one element of this programme, such as a school-based nutrition education project, might be 'to contribute to the reduction of childhood obesity'. A project may have one or two aims. However, to ensure sufficient focus for the project to be effective it is not likely that it will have more than two. A second aim for the project we are using as an example might be to bring about improvements in knowledge about healthy eating among young people in schools.

The objectives should be specific to the project and should set out the concrete outputs of the project. A simple way of thinking about clear objectives is the SMART model. This stands for:

- *specific*: with clear, defined outputs;
- *measurable*: you will be able to know when you have achieved these outputs;
- *agreed*: the outputs are agreed in advance;
- *realistic*: the outputs are not dependent on other factors that are unlikely to happen;
- *time-limited*: the outputs will happen within a set time.

An example of an objective for a healthy eating at schools project could be '1000 children participating in a healthy eating programme in the first year of the project'.

Objectives should contribute directly to the achievement of project aims. A common error in developing objectives is to lose sight of the aims. The link between the aims and the objectives is subject to your invention logic. To return to the example of healthy eating in schools, if you aim to reduce childhood obesity and one of your objectives is to have 1000 children participating in this programme, you need to be clear that healthy eating at school is likely to impact on childhood obesity. To ensure the objectives will contribute to the achievement of the aims, you will need to use your research on the evidence of how previous interventions have worked in similar settings and with similar groups, as discussed in Chapter 3.

Activity 14.2

Imagine you are working in an organization that has identified a high prevalence of cardiovascular disease among south Asian communities in London and you are developing a project to address this. Suggest some draft aims and objectives for the project.

Feedback

You should have reflected on what you have learnt about the difference between a programme aim and a project aim and the difference between an aim and an objective. You need to be clear about how your objectives will contribute to your aim(s) and ensure your objectives are SMART.

Task 5: planning the project's activities

After you have decided on aims and objectives, you need to define the activities that will achieve the objectives. You should include important project management activities, such as the preparation of an interim report for funders. You need to set a timescale for these activities. In doing so, you should remember that some activities will be dependent on the completion of others. It is important to be clear about the interdependence of project activities at this stage because, if one activity is delayed, it may result in the delay of other activities. When you have defined the activities, you need to set 'milestones' for the project. Milestones signal the completion of key activities that indicate progress in the project. They enable you to see easily if the project is, or isn't, on track. A chronogram is a clear way of presenting the project activities and milestones (see Figure 14.1).

When setting a timetable for project activities, you should consider if it is important to include some 'early wins'. Early wins are visible successes at the start of a project that will build commitment to the project from stakeholders.

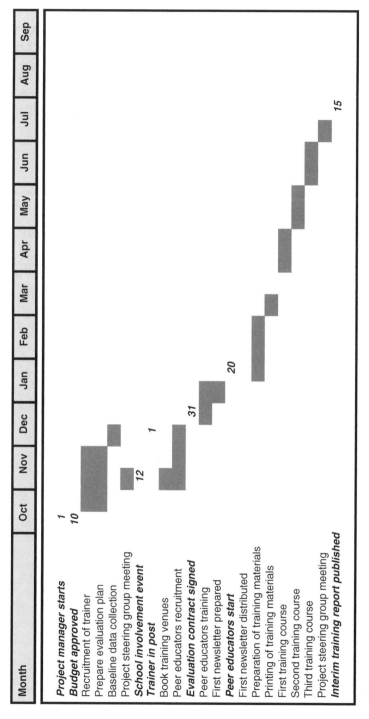

Milestones shown in bold and numbers indicating exact date

Figure 14.1 Chronogram

You need to assign responsibilities for the project activities to the relevant members of the project team, which should ideally be integrated into their work plans to ensure they happen. When developing a work plan it is also important to consider whether the staff member may require any professional development to meet the objectives and to include the method and timescale for meeting these development needs in the work plan.

When planning the project activities, it is essential you include the evaluation of the project. You need to decide what evaluation questions you will seek to answer, what methods you will use and what information you will need. You cannot leave it until the project has started to decide what type of evaluation you will do as by then it may be too late to collect the necessary information. Chapter 15 discusses project evaluations in more detail.

As part of defining the project activities, you need to think about how you will ensure the quality of the project activities and outcomes. There may be internal or external quality standards that are applicable to the project. For example, many agencies have minimum user standards or charters. There may also be legal requirements regarding informed consent or confidentiality.

The type of project monitoring you intend to undertake should also be determined at this stage. Project monitoring information will be required to check the progress of the project and to ensure compliance with applicable quality standards. Monitoring should focus on assessing whether the really key activities are occurring. Data from monitoring may also be used in the overall evaluation of the project. You must be clear about how monitoring information will be collected, who will collect it and who will review it before the implementation of the project proceeds.

You also need to consider what the exit strategy for the project will be. It may be that the nature of the project means that it will come to a definite end at a particular point – for example, if the project is to undertake a piece of research. Alternatively, the project may involve the establishment of a service that will need to be sustained. You need to identify actions you must take to ensure the sustainability of the project at this stage. These could include seeking funding, handing over the project to a different agency or building in income generation.

 Activity 14.3

Based on the aims and objectives you developed in Activity 14.2:

1   Prepare a chronogram of the activities that will achieve the aims and objectives and develop milestones.
2   Develop three 'early wins' for the project.

 Feedback

1 You should have: thought about the activities that will be necessary to ensure you meet each of the objectives; decided what order they need to occur in; identified which

activities are dependent on the completion of other activities; and then developed your milestones.

2 Early wins are visible successes at the start of a project that will build commitment to the project from stakeholders. Some stakeholders may already be committed to the project from its inception but others may require more visible proof of the project's worth before they will commit to it. Some may provide initial commitment but require an early success to maintain that commitment. You should have thought about the type of early wins that can secure this commitment.

Task 6: developing a project budget

A budget is a document that shows how much money you need to carry out the activities required to meet your objectives. It allows you to identify the funding required and how you are proposing to spend it. The budget also enables you to see how much you have actually spent compared to how much you planned to spend and make any necessary adjustments.

A budget breaks down planned expenditure into different categories of expenses often called budget headings or 'account codes'. Examples of budget headings include 'salaries', 'office costs', 'training costs', 'consultancy fees' and 'transport'. Activities are costed separately in a budget and the cost is put in the relevant budget heading or account code. Each agency or funder will have its own account codes. These indicate how the agency breaks down its expenditure in its annual accounts. Generally speaking, the bigger an agency's expenditure the more detailed its account codes will be.

A budget also breaks down planned expenditure into time periods and gives the total cost. Most budgets divide planned expenditure into financial years. However, some budgets may be further broken down into quarters or months.

Figure 14.2 provides an example of a simple budget. A budget needs to contain enough detail for it to be useful in managing the project but not so much detail that it is unwieldy. It is normally drafted by the project coordinator using information provided by members of the project team on the components of the project they will implement. Most organizations have a finance manager who will provide support, test assumptions and critically appraise the draft budget. The project management or steering group, or the relevant finance manager or director for the lead implementing agency, is usually required to approve a draft budget before it becomes final.

The process for developing a budget varies for agency to agency. Generally, the key steps are as follows:

- describe the activities required to reach the project's objectives (see Task 5);
- get information on costs from members of the implementing group or other experts;
- cost the activities and present these costs in the categories of expenses given as budget headings or account codes;
- prepare a budget narrative that describes what the figures are based on.

This is very important. Imagine you come to take over the role of project manager

Costs	Projected Expenditure		
	Year 1	Year 2	Year 3
Total staff costs	*55000*	*56100*	*57222*
Project manager x 1	25000	25500	26010
Secretary x 0.5	10000	10200	10404
Trainer x 1	20000	20400	20808
Total office costs	*7150*	*3938*	*4477*
Office supplies	500	600	800
Office equipment and hardware	4000	500	500
Office rent	1500	1530	1561
Office maintenance and insurance	400	408	416
Communication costs and posted fees	750	900	1200
Total peer educator costs	*15400*	*12400*	*12400*
Recruitment costs	3000	0	0
Consultant to train and support 12 days @ £200 a day	2400	2400	2400
Expenses for peer educators 50 @ £10 a day for 20 days	10000	10000	10000
Total training costs	*7500*	*7500*	*5500*
Training session materials	2500	2500	500
Training room costs 20 days @ £100 a day	2000	2000	2000
Refreshments for training session 20 days @ £50 a day	1000	1000	1000
Creche for training session 20 days @ £100 a day	2000	2000	2000
TOTAL COSTS	**85050**	**79938**	**79599**

Figure 14.2 A simple budget

in the middle of a project. How will you know where the figures come from? You should:

- include a breakdown of global figures;
- include assumptions about beneficiary numbers and consumption;
- include a assumptions about risks;
- include the basis on which you have estimated costs, for example: '4 newsletters at £5,000 each'; 'two part-time peer educators at £10,000' each;
- get finance colleagues to check the draft budget;
- get approval for the draft budget.

The following points are useful tips to help you prepare a budget:

- familiarize yourself with the budget requirements of the funder and lead implementing agency before you start;
- include provision for inflation and other increases where a project continues over several years;
- start as early as possible so you have enough time to involve the project team;
- try to get consensus – it is very difficult to manage a budget if some of the people involved say they never agreed the costs in the budget;
- label different drafts of the budget clearly and if you circulate them to colleagues, keep track of the master copy;
- do not change costs without consulting the person who gave them to you or you may find you misunderstood what the costs were based on and are left with insufficient funding in the budget;
- ask for technical advice – you cannot know what everything costs.

Once you have developed the budget, you need to secure the necessary funding. Funding may be available from within the overall budget of the lead implementing agency or from a national government programme of which the project forms part. Alternatively, it may be necessary to raise money for the project from grant-giving bodies, commissioning agencies, trusts or partner organizations. Increasingly, health promotion projects tend to be funded by a variety of different sources with a single project often receiving funds from government, partner organizations and trusts.

 Activity 14.4

Imagine you are the project manager for a two-year project focusing on a health promotion issue of your choice that involves providing training sessions, developing media advocacy and undertaking research, and which will employ a project manager, a secretary, two training coordinators and a researcher. Think about the types of costs that might be involved and design a budget.

 Feedback

Reflect on what you have learnt about the purpose of a budget and how it is used. Think about what level of detail you will need to ensure you can compare actual expenditure to planned expenditure as the project progresses. Make sure you only group similar types of expenses together – for example, do not combine salary with non-salary costs.

Decide on and divide the budget into equal time periods. These could be each year or each quarter. Show the total for the two years clearly. Decide on whether you need to include an increase in costs in the second year for inflation.

Task 7: identify assumptions and risks

Every project involves making assumptions and taking risks. The important thing is to understand what these are and to manage them.

Assumptions are factors outside the control of the project that will negatively impact on the project if they are not met. If an assumption is not met, other action will need to be taken. This action should be identified in advance. For example, the availability of healthy food locally is an assumption. If it is not available locally, it will need to be brought in from further away which may affect the cost of the project.

A risk is a potential hazard, in effect a critical assumption. If a risk is allowed to manifest, the success of the project will be threatened. Therefore, action needs to be taken to minimize risks and this should be built into the project plan. Potential risks include lack of or withdrawal of funding, insufficient support from key stakeholders and failure to recruit to a crucial project post. Action to minimize these risks could include early and ongoing involvement of key stakeholders, including funders, and working with partner organizations to secure secondments for crucial posts. If a risk is identified that is likely to be realized because no action can be taken to minimize it, the project should be redesigned.

 Activity 14.5

Imagine you are working on a project to reduce smoking among teenage girls using peer education in schools. What might the assumptions and risks be? What action might you take to minimize the risks?

 Feedback

There would be a number of assumptions and risk with such a project. For example, the project would require the participation of schools and there is a risk that headteachers may not wish their schools to become involved. This risk could be minimized by early consultation with headteachers and their inclusion in the project steering group.

Task 8: getting approval for the project plan

Before you proceed with the implementation of the project, you need to get approval for the project plan. The type of approval you need will depend on where the funding for the project is coming from, the type of organization that is the lead agency and whether the project has a project management or steering group. It may be necessary to get formal or statutory approvals for the project plan. It is also important to give stakeholders involved in developing the project plan an opportunity to feed back on it even if their approval is not formally required. Stakeholders are much more likely actively to support a project if they feel ownership of it.

Implementing the project

Task 1: undertaking defined activities and monitoring progress

The project manager may be responsible for undertaking many of the project activities. However, as you have learnt, health promotion programmes are increasingly delivered by partnerships where different individuals and organizations take responsibility for project activities. A partnership approach to project implementation can strengthen a project's capacity, in that the resources of more than one organization are available. However, it also creates more potential for delay, in that partner organizations' capacities and priorities may change and individuals may move on to new roles.

Therefore, it is very important that the project manager is actively monitoring progress with the implementation of activities, paying particular attention to those activities on which others are dependent and the assumptions and risks identified in the project plan. Line managers of staff members working on the project should undertake regular performance review meetings with these staff and ensure that information on any delay or problem identified and action to resolve this is fed back to the project manager. The project manager should also monitor whether the assumptions identified in the project plan are proving correct and that the risks are not being realized. Using a chronogram (see Figure 14.1) and setting milestones for the project will help monitor progress.

Task 2: collecting information

The project manager and other members of the project team should seek new information that may be relevant to the project throughout its implementation. This could include: new research; changes in national priorities or strategies; and information concerning the failures or successes of similar projects. Information may come from professional journals, national or local health promotion forums and visits to other projects.

Task 3: approving expenditure and budget monitoring

The overall financial management of health promotion projects will usually be the responsibility of the finance department of the lead implementing agency. However, the project manager is likely to have some specific responsibilities.

One such responsibility is the approval of expenditure related to the project. The form of this approval varies from organization to organization but usually it is the signing off of a written form. Approving an expense involves checking it is included in the project budget and that it costs no more than the amount provided for this in the budget. If an expense is incurred which is not provided for in the project budget or which exceeds budget provision, the budget-holder may need to get approval from the financial manager to go ahead.

Another financial management responsibility is that of reviewing actual expenditure to date as compared to the budget. This may need to be done quarterly or annually, depending on the requirements of the lead implementing agency or funder. It is important to bear in mind that some project expenditure may occur regularly throughout the project, for example salaries and rent, whereas other large items of expenditure may occur only once, for example equipment purchase or building works. If regular or large payments are delayed, it will have a significant impact on the overall project expenditure. Differences between the budget and actual expenditure are sometimes known as budget variances or slippage.

Budget variances can impact on the availability of funds as some funders may offer funds on the condition that they are spent within a set time period. In addition, some funders may specify in detail what their funds can be spent on so if one project activity is delayed, it should not be assumed that funds can be diverted for another project activity. It is important to check any conditions attached to funding before implementing the project.

Task 4: making changes to the project plan as necessary

It may be necessary to change the project plan. Changes could include adjustments to project activities dependent on what is working so far, any new research or assumptions not being met. Changes could also include amendments to the timetable because some activities have taken longer than planned so other things cannot start on time. It may also be necessary to make adjustments regarding who is responsible for certain activities because of changes in the capacity or commitment or partner agencies, or because new agencies become involved. Finally, it may be necessary to make revisions to the budget based on changes to costs or as a result of delays in project activities.

Any changes to the project plan may need to be approved, depending on their size and importance, and the management structure of the project.

Task 5: reporting progress

The project manager should report regularly on the project's progress to different audiences. Progress reporting fulfils a number of different and important functions. First, it enables the project team to deliver the project activities for which they are responsible. Second, it provides accountability to the project management or steering group. Third, it maintains and builds commitment and ownership among stakeholders. Fourth, it keeps users and potential beneficiaries informed and can encourage their involvement. Fifth, it shares information on the project's progress and lessons learnt to those who could benefit from this, such as those working on similar projects. Finally, reporting on and advertising the project's progress will be important for its sustainability.

Completing the project

Task 1: evaluating whether the project achieved its objectives

You need to assess to what extent the project has achieved its aims and objectives it set itself and answer the evaluation questions you set for the project. This is discussed in more detail in Chapter 15.

Task 2: staff appraisal

Line managers of staff working on the project need to undertake regular performance review meetings with staff throughout the course of the project. Formal feedback on performance needs to be provided to staff in the form of a staff appraisal annually and at the completion of the project. Staff members should be given the opportunity to say how they think they performed as part of the appraisal. The project manager may be taking on a new role after the completion of the project. It is essential they undertake staff appraisals before they move on.

Task 3: handing the project over or finishing the project

You should have identified any necessary action to ensure the project's sustainability when you planned the project's activities. Depending on the nature of the project, it may be handed over to another organization for continuation. Handing over the project will involve inducting the new staff, explaining the management of premises and taking steps to ensure continuity of service.

Alternatively, if the project was by nature of a fixed term or if it has achieved its objectives, its purpose may have been achieved and it is now finished. Finishing a project will itself require some action depending on the nature of the project. For example, a research project may involve the production and presentation of a report of the research. Alternatively, finishing a project may necessitate the disposal of assets, terminating staff contracts and making arrangements for other agencies to take over any residual functions.

Task 4: producing a final project report

The final task of project management will usually be the production of a final report. A final report may be required by a project funder or the lead implementing agency, in which case the format of the report will generally be specified. Final reports usually include the following sections:

*   achievements of the project (with reference to the evaluation);
*   failures and the reasons for them;
*   lessons learnt during the implementation of the project;

- resources used by the project;
- partner agencies;
- steps taken to complete the project;
- future action identified;
- financial report including a breakdown of expenditure, the source of funding and an explanation of variances from the budget.

Even if a final report is not formally required, it may be useful to produce one in order to ensure that the information developed in the course of the project is not lost when the project manager and others involved move on to different roles.

Summary

A project management approach should improve the efficiency and effectiveness of health promotion delivery. Project management can be broken down into project planning, project implementation and project completion. Each of these stages involves several interrelated tasks.

References

Beachamp DE, Childress JF (1999) *New Ethics for the Public's Health*. Oxford: Oxford University Press.
Scally G (2001) Project management, in the *Oxford Handbook of Public Health Practice*. Oxford: Oxford University Press.
Speller V (1998) *Quality, Evidence and Effectiveness in Health Promotion*. London: Routledge.
Tones K, Green J (2004) *Health Promotion: Planning and strategies*. London: Sage.

Further reading

Ewles L, Simnett E (2003) *Promoting Health: A practical guide*. London: Ballière Tindall.
Naidoo J, Wills J (2000) *Health Promotion: Foundations for practice*. London: Ballière Tindall.

Overview

This chapter considers the evaluation of health promotion, drawing examples from sexual health. It discusses the importance of evaluation and of setting the right evaluation questions. It then considers different evaluation designs and methods of data collection. Finally the chapter identifies some pitfalls to avoid in evaluating health promotion.

Learning objectives

After reading this chapter, you will be better able to:

- **explain the purpose of evaluation and define evaluation questions**
- **select the best design and methods to answer these questions**
- **avoid pitfalls in evaluation**

Key terms

Evaluation The critical assessment of the value of an activity.

Formative evaluation An evaluation aiming to refine the process by which an intervention is delivered.

Outcomes measures Change in status as a result of the system processes (in the health services context, the change in health status as a result of care).

Process The use of resources or the activity within a system.

Summative evaluation An evaluation aiming to establish the value of an intervention.

Defining evaluation questions

Outcomes

Those funding, planning, delivering or receiving health promotion are entitled to ask questions about these services, the obvious one being, does the intervention achieve its aims? Most health promotion aims primarily to prevent diseases or other biological outcomes, some of which, such as obesity, are associated with disease, while others, such as teenage pregnancy, are regarded as negative for other reasons. Some interventions aim to promote health in a positive sense, such as fitness or autonomy. Whether or not negative outcomes are prevented or positive outcomes achieved will have important consequences for those experiencing the intervention and those funding and delivering it. It is therefore important to identify whether or not interventions are effective, and this cannot be assumed (Bonell *et al.* 2003).

Some view health promotion as aiming only to empower individuals to enact the behaviours that they desire rather than to bring about the behaviours that health promoters desire. This view is expressed for example in Chapter 1. The logical corollary of this is that evaluation should focus on whether 'needs' (e.g. for information or for skills) which are required to enable empowerment are met or not, rather than whether behaviours change or biological outcomes are influenced. We would disagree with this approach for two reasons. First, many interventions aim not to empower but to influence behaviours directly, for example by means such as tobacco taxes and seatbelt laws, and therefore cannot be assessed in terms of meeting needs. Second, our information on what needs are key to addressing particular health issues will always be incomplete and may often be inaccurate. If evaluations only evaluate whether apparent 'needs' have been met they will not identify instances where interventions have successfully met 'needs' but have had no effects on behaviours because the 'needs' addressed are not in fact key influences on behaviour or other 'needs' must also be met to influence behaviour.

Processes

Questions may be asked about the process of implementing or receiving an intervention as well as its effectiveness. They can explore why an intervention was or wasn't effective and how easy it might be to undertake it in another context. A process evaluation can ask:

- What does the intervention entail?
- Is the intervention feasible to deliver in a specific setting by a specific provider?
- Does the intervention reach those it is intended to?
- Is the intervention acceptable to providers, recipients and other stakeholders?
- Is the intervention likely to prove as feasible and acceptable and have as high coverage in other contexts?

Process evaluations should describe how interventions are planned and implemented in enough detail so that providers elsewhere can judge whether and how to reproduce the intervention. In many cases, published evaluations provide rigorous evidence on effectiveness but little information on the intervention itself (Ellis *et al.* 2003).

Acceptability is an important criterion of judgement for interventions, not merely as a predictor of likely effectiveness but in its own terms. Even if an intervention is effective, it should only be implemented more widely if it is also acceptable to those receiving it. For example, even if an intervention was found to be effective in reducing HIV transmission among gay men by criminalizing sex between men, it would not be acceptable to them and so should not be implemented.

Although evaluations can explore effectiveness and process together, sometimes the priority will be to explore intervention process only. For example, with a new intervention, the priority may be to explore how the intervention can be refined. An intervention that is not very feasible or acceptable, or which has poor coverage, is unlikely to be very effective. Evaluations geared towards refinement are termed 'formative' evaluations. Once the intervention is refined, an outcome evaluation can be undertaken. This would be a 'summative' evaluation; i.e. establishing whether or not the intervention is effective. There are numerous cases of interventions found in outcome evaluations to be ineffective because of problems with process which could have been solved had the intervention been subject to preliminary formative evaluation (Elford *et al.* 2000).

A process-only evaluation might also be required in the case of an intervention found effective in one or more settings being transferred to a new setting. While the generalizability of effectiveness of an intervention from one setting to another can never be guaranteed, those implementing the intervention in the new setting might decide that if the intervention is found to be feasible, is reaching its targets and is acceptable in the new setting, then they can be reasonably confident that the intervention will be effective there as well. They may therefore decide to invest in a process-only evaluation.

Evaluations examine intervention processes and outcomes in a particular setting. Unless they can guide work in other settings they are unlikely to be worth the money invested in them. The overall purpose of evaluation should be to inform the deployment of feasible, accessible, acceptable and effective (and/or cost-effective) interventions in new settings in which these effects are likely to be repeated, and to prevent the deployment of interventions that are ineffective or harmful. To maximize the extent to which they achieve this, evaluations need to explore how local contextual factors influenced the feasibility of delivery.

Choosing the best evaluation design

Evaluation design refers to the overall structure and logic of the evaluation. Issues to be considered include whether evaluations should employ comparison as well as intervention groups, how participants will be allocated to these, how sampling will occur and what sorts of measures will be used. Design differs from methods, which refer to how data are actually collected.

Although the questions set out in the above section are obviously important, choosing the design that best answers them is not; controversy rages about the merits of different designs. The following section discusses the main elements of a rigorous evaluation, first of outcomes then of processes.

Outcome evaluation

Outcome evaluations aim to examine the effects of interventions on recipients. Interventions should have clear aims with agreed outcomes and evaluations should if possible involve a comparison group.

Clear aims and agreed outcomes

If an evaluation is to demonstrate that an intervention has achieved its aims of preventing or promoting certain negative or positive outcomes, its aims must be agreed and stated. Funders, providers and potential recipients should have a say in identifying these aims. Once aims have been set, appropriate outcome measures can be identified. Outcomes measures are indicators that are used to measure whether aims have been achieved. An outcome evaluation will measure rates of the outcomes among those who experience the intervention. Sometimes, especially in the case of the prevention of relatively uncommon outcomes, proxies for the outcome are measured, rather than, or in addition to, the outcomes themselves. For example, a proxy for teenage pregnancy might be sexual debut before age 16 (Wellings *et al.* 2001). Sometimes biological outcome information will be collected directly, for example by testing saliva samples for HIV infection. However it is more common for information about biological or behavioural outcomes to be collected using questionnaire surveys, which are discussed below.

Evaluators must state what the outcomes are (and how these relate to the intervention aims) *before* analysis commences and report on *all* of these outcomes. This is termed 'pre-hypothesization' of outcomes. Evaluators should not merely report on outcome measures that show a significant positive effect and neglect to report on those which showed no effect or a negative effect. Nor should evaluators search their results for any significant positive outcome and report this, even though they had not stated at outset that they would be examining this particular outcome. This is known as 'data-dredging' and leads to reporting bias.

A comparison group

Effectiveness is relative not absolute. For example, if we found that the rate of unintended pregnancy among young people who had experienced a sex education intervention was 20 per 1000, it would be difficult to judge whether the intervention was a success or not. What we need to know is how many unintended pregnancies there would have been if the intervention had not occurred. This would still be true if we knew the unintended pregnancy rate before and after the intervention. We might, for example, find that before an intervention the rate of unintended pregnancies is 10 per 1000 and that, after it, the rate is 20 per 1000. This might seem to suggest ineffectiveness. However, if we were to learn that the rate would have risen from 10 to 30 per 1000 had the young people not experienced the intervention, we might consider the intervention effective. Ideally, to identify whether or not an intervention is effective, the outcomes experienced by those receiving the intervention must be compared to similar people who have not received it.

'Before and after' evaluations are not an optimal study design because they don't account for changes in outcome measures that arise for reasons other than the intervention (Oakley 1990). Outcome rates can change because of secular trends or because of age. In some cases, those accessing an intervention, such as sexually transmitted infection counselling, are doing so because they are behaving more riskily than they usually do, and their behaviour then returns to its typical level for reasons unconnected with the intervention (Stephenson and Imrie 1998).

Therefore, if possible, outcome evaluations should involve the measurement of outcomes among an 'intervention' group and a 'comparison' group, who usually receive standard care rather than the new intervention. Such designs are 'experimental' and sometimes referred to as 'trials'. Fair comparison of outcomes requires that the two groups are composed of similar sorts of people, otherwise these other differences, and not the intervention, might explain differences in outcomes. This is known as confounding. Although statisticians can adjust for some confounding effects, these adjustments cannot be perfect and ensuring the comparability of groups at the outset is preferable.

One way to promote comparability is to use a 'matched' comparison design. Here, efforts are made to identify people's attributes that may influence outcomes and ensure that the groups contain similar numbers of people with these attributes. For instance, groups can be matched on socioeconomic status, HIV prevalence etc. The problem with this approach is that not all the attributes that influence an outcome will be known. Many factors can influence people's actions and it will never be possible to identify all these. Since groups cannot be matched according to all such factors, random allocation of people to intervention or to comparison group in a randomized controlled trial (RCT) is a better way to ensure these groups are similar. Randomization of enough people distributes factors that influence the outcomes, known and unknown, equally between intervention and comparison groups (Gotzsche *et al.* 1997). Evaluations with comparison groups should report on the baseline profiles of each, especially in terms of potentially confounding factors, to check for any significant differences so that if possible these can be adjusted for statistically.

Some argue it is unethical to use comparison groups in evaluations because participants in these groups are denied the intervention. This argument assumes that the intervention in question would benefit participants. However, if a state of 'equipoise' exists, i.e. there is uncertainty about whether participants would benefit or be harmed by being in one group rather than another, it is ethical to undertake such an evaluation (Oakley 1990). In order to be ethical, trials need to ensure that those in comparison groups are not denied care that they otherwise would receive if they were not involved in a trial.

Health promotion evaluators shouldn't automatically opt for individual-randomized trials of the sort generally used in clinical trials, where individuals are allocated to receive or not receive the intervention in question, without first considering whether a cluster-randomized trial would be more appropriate. The latter allocate clusters of people (schools, communities etc.) rather than individuals to receive an intervention or not. People's health is influenced by their social and physical environment as well as by their behaviour and some health promotion interventions attempt to influence such factors. Even interventions that don't aim to bring about 'environmental' effects may have 'added value' resulting from whole groups of people interacting in new ways as a result of receiving an intervention. Individual, as opposed to cluster allocation studies, cannot examine such effects. Cluster-based evaluations are also less affected by 'contamination', another methodological problem that can beset evaluations (Torgerson 2001). Contamination occurs where individuals not allocated to receive the intervention actually do so indirectly via their contact with people receiving it. Contamination results in underestimation of intervention effects. Although it can be adjusted for statistically, this is imperfect. Cluster evaluations are generally less prone to contamination because people usually interact less with those from other clusters.

Where randomization is impossible, matched comparison designs are preferable to studies either that don't have any comparison groups or those that involve an unmatched comparison group. Where interventions, such as mass media campaigns, can only be provided across entire populations, comparison groups cannot be set up and the only option is to undertake an observational 'before and after' evaluation.

All outcome evaluations, whether 'before and after' or comparative, require quantitative data on outcomes to be collected from fairly large samples of people to maximize the likelihood that any apparent differences either between baseline and follow-up measures, or between intervention and comparison group measures, aren't merely the result of chance. Statisticians can undertake 'power calculations' about what size samples are required to show what effects in specific populations.

Process evaluation

Exploration of a diversity of perspectives

Process evaluations examine intervention planning, delivery and receipt in order to explore whether an intervention is feasible, reaches those it is intended to and is acceptable. Process evaluations should assess how views on feasibility, coverage and acceptability differ among different sorts of people. For example, most providers might think an intervention is feasible but those at the very front line of delivery may not, and might have some ideas about how to make it more feasible. An intervention might be acceptable to all who receive it except for one sub-group who find it completely unacceptable. This is important to know.

Use of qualitative and quantitative data

Quantitative data is essential in assessing factors such as extent of delivery, coverage of target groups and level of satisfaction. Qualitative data is essential in building up a richer picture of what went well and what went less well, and the importance of the particularities of provider, context and participant in determining this. Whereas the aim of quantitative research is identifying statistically significant associations, the purpose of qualitative research is to develop theory about social processes by clarifying how different people view the world, what concepts they use to do this and how they relate different concepts to each other. Because of this, qualitative research does not need to involve samples that are 'powered' to examine significance but rather needs to involve samples that are diverse in terms of social position, identity and perspective.

Activity 15.1

The Minister of Health wants to reduce rates of chlamydia among teenagers. The testing and treatment for chlamydia is currently provided for free by local sexual health clinics; however, rates of use by teens are low. There is an idea that offering services in local youth projects would reduce rates, because more teenagers would go for testing and treatment there.

1 What sort of research questions would an evaluation of youth project-based services need to ask?
2 What study design would be best for answering these questions?

 Feedback

1 The main evaluation questions might be:

- Is offering services testing for and treating chlamydia in youth projects a more effective way of reducing prevalence than offering services in sexual health clinics only?
- Are young people more comfortable going to youth project-based services?
- How many and who are using youth project-based services compared with sexual health clinics?
- What do service providers and youth project workers think about the new provision?

2 The study design to answer these questions most appropriately would be a cluster RCT with integral process evaluation. This would allow for rigorous examination of effectiveness (this could include overall rates, as well as proxy measures such as uptake of testing and treatment) and would also provide information on the acceptability and accessibility of the youth services testing and treatment services.

 Activity 15.2

1 A review of existing rigorous outcome evaluations found that postnatal home visiting programmes were effective in reducing rates of postnatal depression. All of the programmes in the review were based in the USA. You are about to set up a similar intervention in the UK. What are the main evaluation questions?
2 What evaluation design could you carry out to identify the challenges that may be faced when initiating home visiting programmes across the UK?

 Feedback

1 The main evaluation questions might be:

- Is it feasible to deliver such a programme in the UK?
- Can the programme reach the women targeted?
- What do service providers and the women targeted think of the programme?
- What aspects of the programme need to be changed to maximize the success of the programmes in the UK compared with in the USA?
- What contextual factors influence feasibility, coverage and acceptability?

2 You could carry out a process-only evaluation. Ideally this would involve the implementation of a pilot programme in one area before national roll-out. The evaluation
would explore the experiences of those using the programme, those planning and
running the programme and other key stakeholders. It would also collect quantitative
data on coverage and acceptability of the programme among sub-groups of women.
If you wanted to measure the effectiveness of the programme in a UK context, you
would need to consider running an RCT.

Using the appropriate methods

Data can be collected in different ways. Choice of method depends on the type of
evaluation design to be used as well as practical considerations relating to the
characteristics of the people involved and the resources available to the evaluation.
These aspects will be discussed further under each method below. These methods
can be used separately or in combination.

Surveys

Surveys involve asking a number of preset questions in a standard way to relatively
large numbers of participants. Surveys can be self-completed by participants using
questionnaires or participants can engage in structured interviews with researchers.
'Closed' questions have a predefined set of answer options, to provide quantitative
data, whereas 'open' questions allow the participant to give an answer in their own
words, usually to provide qualitative data.

Surveys can be used to explore outcomes or processes. For instance, in the
evaluation of a mass-media smoking cessation campaign, a survey might examine
outcomes by asking questions about knowledge of the effects of smoking on
health, current smoking behaviours or health status. To examine process, it may
explore people's awareness of or views on the campaign. Surveys usually provides
simple answers to questions; useful for quantifying an issue but not for providing
in-depth information about it (e.g. exploring why people start to think about
quitting or their views on how the campaign influenced them).

Evaluators need to take into account the circumstances of their potential participants when planning a survey. Literacy problems or other factors may impede
the use of self-completion questionnaires and therefore necessitate structured
interview surveys. However, the latter will be more time-consuming. Even surveys
relying on self-completion questionnaires still require considerable time and
staffing resources for the design, production, distribution and collection of
questionnaires, as well as data input and analysis.

Semi-structured interviews

A key evaluation method for gathering in-depth information is interviewing,
where a member of the evaluation team engages in a 'conversation' with an inter-

viewee that is less structured than the sorts of structured interviews discussed above. The interviewer asks questions but does not restrict the interviewee to answering according to preset options and allows the participant considerable leeway in guiding the course of the interchange. The interviewer can probe or introduce new questions when it is felt that more information on a certain topic would be useful. This allows for the collection of qualitative data and a more in-depth exploration of the interviewee's experiences and perceptions. Interviews can be used to gather in-depth data about outcomes but are more often used to explore people's experiences and views on process. Data from semi-structured interviews is not used to quantify but rather to describe and explain.

Interviews are semi-structured, in which the interviewer has a specific topic-guide used to steer the discussion around set themes, using probes if necessary. Interviews are audio- or video-recorded and transcribed, or written notes are taken. In some cases, it may be essential that interviews are conducted by someone who the interviewee can identify with, for example someone of the same age, gender or ethnicity. In other cases it may be that differences in identity are acceptable or even potentially more useful or acceptable to interviewees. Interview-based research is usually very time-consuming but does not involve such great production or distribution costs as survey research.

Focus group discussions

Focus group discussions are another method for gathering in-depth, qualitative data from a relatively small number of participants. Rather than interviewing one person at a time, a group of approximately 6 to 12 people are brought together and asked questions, again in a semi- or unstructured way. Rather than exploring individual views in depth as interviews do, focus groups allow a group of peers to share their views and allow the researchers to observe group interaction. This method can be used to examine social norms and ways that these can influence attitudes and behaviours (though it cannot measure behaviour itself). Combining focus group and interview data can enable evaluators to compare different points of view, different motivations and the degree of consensus on a topic. Focus groups should not be regarded merely as a time-saving way to interview lots of people; the questions that can be answered by each method are different. Although running a focus group may not take much time, they are usually very time-consuming to organize beforehand and to transcribe and analyse afterwards. Although people sometimes feel more comfortable in discussing certain topics when talking among their peers rather than on their own in an interview, sometimes they do not. Evaluators should be aware of: cultural sensitivities about discussing certain issues in a group setting; power relations within groups whereby the views of some dominate those of others; confidentiality; and difficulties in setting up groups across widely dispersed populations. Like interviews, focus groups are most commonly used to explore process.

Like interviews, focus groups can be audio- or video-recorded or notes taken. It is helpful for two research team members to be present; one to facilitate the discussion and the other to observe interaction.

Activity 15.3

You want to carry out a process evaluation of a peer education intervention to promote HIV prevention and sexual health among gay men. In this evaluation you want to explore whether the intervention was delivered as planned, who it reached, and how acceptable it was to the peer educators, their peers and those planning and training the peer educators. What methods would be most appropriate to use?

 Feedback

A variety of methodological options are available to you. You might consider using a combination of the following methods:

- questionnaire completed by peer educators (asking how confident they felt in delivering peer education; how motivated; their perception of the intervention – what worked well, what was hard, what would have helped)
- this could be supplemented with individual semi-structured interviews with the peer educators or focus group discussions with them
- interviews with trainers of peer educators and planners of the programme (how did they feel the training went; challenges to delivering it; perception of how peer educators received training and accepted new role)
- focus groups with recipients of peer education to explore their experiences of receiving the intervention

Common problems in evaluating health promotion interventions

Being over-ambitious

It is tempting to want to carry out the most comprehensive evaluation possible, targeting a number of research questions and incorporating a sophisticated design with multiple methods. Although this may be entirely appropriate for some interventions, for others this can be a case of 'too much, too soon'. A complex and large-scale evaluation can be expensive to carry out and will require staff and infrastructure to do so effectively. It is important to weigh up the resources available to you with the questions you want to be answered.

Attempting to carry out an over-ambitious evaluation can, in some circumstances, mean that the evaluation will need to be aborted because there are not enough resources to complete it. It is far more sensible to be 'up front' from the outset with the funders of research, programme directors and other decision-makers about the capacity for evaluation and the types of appropriate research questions that can be answered regarding the intervention. As discussed earlier, sometimes the priority should be to do a relatively simple process evaluation well, rather than a complex outcome evaluation badly.

Trying to evaluate your own programme

High-quality evaluation of an intervention *can* be carried out by the staff who deliver the intervention under evaluation. However, this can be very challenging for several reasons. Those implementing a programme may not have the time or skills to organize, as well as carry out, an evaluation. Also, by evaluating your own programme, others may fear the evaluation has been biased by the staff's own desire for the programme to do well. Given these problems, it can be very useful to recruit specialized staff or commission a specialist agency to design and manage an evaluation. This can help avoid bias and/or the suspicion of bias and ensures that the evaluation is given the attention it needs by individuals with appropriate skills.

Involving evaluators too late in the process

Planning and carrying out an evaluation late in the development of a programme can limit the scope of the questions the evaluation can ask. For example, if the main purpose of the evaluation is to learn how individuals and communities have changed because of an intervention, it would not be possible to do this if the evaluation was not in place before the intervention was underway because no 'baseline' measures can be taken. In such a scenario, one solution is to evaluate intervention process rather than outcomes. Alternatively, it might be possible to delay an evaluation of outcomes until the intervention in question is rolled out to a new area.

Forgetting the importance of ethical issues

Informed consent

Participants should only be involved in an intervention *and* the evaluation (including what and how data will be collected and used) on the basis of their prior, informed consent. Where individuals are allocated randomly to intervention or comparison group, this should also be done only after participants have given informed consent. The information provided should be clear and easy for potential participants to understand and they should be given the opportunity to ask questions. Issues of confidentiality should be explained. It should be made clear that participants' consent is voluntary and that they can choose to withdraw at any time during the evaluation. Even in situations where it is not practical for participation in the intervention to be voluntary (e.g. participation in mass-media campaigns delivered within a cluster RCT), participants should still be asked for their voluntary, informed consent to participate in data collection for the evaluation.

Storage and use of data

The storage of data that may contain sensitive and confidential information should be considered before data collection. Information that personally identifies individuals should be kept separate from their process and outcome data. For example, each participant may be assigned a code that is used to identify their questionnaires or interview transcripts, rather than their name. Any contact details provided by participants should be kept separately and all data should be stored securely. Finally, data must be reported both accurately and transparently. When reporting, data should be anonymized sufficiently so that individuals cannot be identified from their responses. Where this anonymity is not possible, the individuals should be given the opportunity to vet their responses to ensure they are happy for them to be made public.

 Activity 15.4

Using a cluster RCT with integral process evaluation, you are evaluating an intervention that aims to prevent teenage pregnancy in intervention schools by improving teachers' skills in delivering sex education and training school nurses to offer one-to-one sexual health advice. Rates of teenage pregnancy are then compared with non-intervention schools where sex education is provided but where no additional training is provided to teachers or school nurses. Consider what arrangements you need to make for gaining informed consent for participation in the intervention and in the evaluation. Sex education is compulsory in all schools.

 Feedback

You cannot seek the informed consent of students for their involvement in sex education because this is compulsory both in intervention and comparison schools. However, you must gain the informed consent of students for their involvement in data collection. You must also obtain the informed consent of other individuals, such as teachers and nurses, for involvement in data collection. Ethics committees will generally require that parents should also be asked for their consent for their children's participation in the evaluation. You cannot seek the individual consent of students for their allocation to intervention or comparison group because allocation is on a cluster rather than an individual basis. Seeking the informed consent of the headteacher (as 'leader' of the cluster) should not be thought of as an adequate alternative to individual student consent to allocation. However, practically it will be necessary to secure their informed consent if the evaluation is to be feasible. This must be done prior to any allocation if the trial is to be unbiased.

Summary

Evaluation is necessary to examine not only the outcomes but also the process of planning, delivery and receipt of interventions. The optimal design to examine the *effectiveness* of health promotion will generally be the RCT. This can have an integral process evaluation to examine feasibility, coverage and acceptability and how these are influenced by context. Process-only evaluations can be useful to refine new interventions or examine potential transferability of established interventions. Evaluations can collect data via methods such as surveys, interviews and focus groups. Pitfalls to avoid in undertaking evaluations include being over-ambitious, trying to evaluate your own intervention, undertaking an evaluation too late and neglecting ethical responsibilities.

References

Bonell CP, Bennett R, Oakley A (2003) Sexual health should be subject to experimental evaluation, in J Stephenson, J Imrie, C Bonell (eds) *Effective Sexual Health Interventions: Issues in experimental evaluation.* Oxford: Oxford University Press.

Elford J, Bolding G, Sherr L (2000) Peer education has no significant impact on HIV risk behaviours among gay men in London. *AIDS*, 15(4): 535–8.

Ellis S, Barnett-Page E, Morgan A, Taylor L, Walters R, Goodrich J (2003) *HIV Prevention: A review of reviews assessing the effectiveness of interventions to reduce the risk of sexual transmission.* London: Health Development Agency.

Oakley A (1990) Who's afraid of the randomised controlled trial? in H Roberts (ed.) *Women's Health Counts.* London: Routledge.

Stephenson J, Imrie J (1998) Why do we need randomized controlled trials to assess behavioural interventions? *British Medical Journal*, 316: 611–13.

Torgerson C (2001) Contamination in trials: is cluster randomization the answer? *British Medical Journal*, 322: 355–7.

Wellings K, Nanchahal K, Macdowall W, McManus S, Erens B, Mercer C, Johnson A, Copas A, Korovessis C, Fenton K, Field J (2001) Sexual behaviour in Britain: early heterosexual experience. *Lancet*, 358: 1843–9.

16 Transfer and scale-up of health promotion interventions

Overview

In this chapter you will learn about the transfer of healthy promotion interventions previously undertaken in one site to other sites. You will consider the extent to which interventions found effective in one site can be assumed to be so in another and whether transferred interventions will be feasible, acceptable, achieve adequate coverage and address key needs. You will then consider how interventions can be scaled up from pilots to full-scale implementation and the decisions that should be made to maximize the likely success of scale-up. The chapter draws examples from HIV prevention to illustrate the points made. The arguments made are equally relevant to interventions aiming to prevent other diseases or to promote health in a positive sense.

Learning objectives

After reading this chapter, you will be better able to:

- explain the factors that are likely to influence whether an intervention found effective in one site might be so in another
- describe how feasibility, coverage and acceptability will vary between sites and what contextual factors will affect this
- explain how interventions must address the key needs of populations if they are to be effective
- describe how health promotion interventions can be transferred from one site to another
- describe the process of scaling up interventions and the factors that will influence the success of moving from a pilot to full-scale implementation

Key terms

Coverage The extent to which an intervention is received by those it targets.

Fidelity The extent to which a subsequent implementation of an intervention is faithful in terms of the process of delivery to how the intervention was implemented in the original site.

Modification A planned process of altering an intervention to ensure it maximally addresses health promotion needs and is feasible, achieves adequate coverage and is acceptable in a new site of implementation.

Normative need The capacity for a population to benefit from a health promotion intervention.

Pilot An initial, small-scale implementation of an intervention accompanied by an evaluation of its process and/or outcomes.

Scale-up The implementation of an intervention previously provided in the context of a pilot across a wider area and/or to a broader population.

Sustainability The extent to which an intervention may be continued beyond its initial implementation; this may be dependent upon a continued source of funding, programme effectiveness or changing priorities.

Transferability The extent to which the results of a study as it applies to a particular patient group or setting hold true for another population or context.

Transfer of health promotion interventions from one site to another

Most health promoters would prefer to deploy interventions that have already been 'tried and tested' elsewhere rather than 'reinventing the wheel' in their own context. Most evaluators would see their role as informing the deployment of feasible, accessible, acceptable and effective interventions in other sites and not merely promoting the success of interventions in the sites in which they were evaluated. However, both groups would recognize that most health promotion interventions cannot be transferred from one site to another without modifying them to a lesser or greater extent to ensure they fit the new context.

The need for modification is generally greater with health promotion interventions than with biomedical interventions, such as surgical procedures or pharmacological treatments. The reason for this lies in the fact that the mechanisms of action of health promotion interventions overwhelmingly involve social processes, such as verbal and non-verbal communication. How communication proceeds and what affects it are hugely dependent on local social structures and culture. In contrast, the *main* mechanisms of action of, for example, surgical and pharmacological interventions, are biological. The effects of biomedical interventions will sometimes vary because of biological differences between populations (e.g. as a result of differences in vulnerability to disease or response to treatments between men and women or between different ethnic groups). Surgical and pharmacological interventions are also delivered via social processes, such as consultations, referrals etc., so that there may need to be some modification of these between sites. However, overall, it is likely that between-site variation will be much less with biomedical than with health promotion interventions. Thus, while surgical and pharmacological interventions that are effective among women in London might, as long as they are delivered appropriately, be expected to be effective among men in Lusaka too, a health promotion intervention that is effective among women in San Francisco cannot be assumed to be so – without modification – among men in Soweto. The next section considers in more detail the factors that influence whether an intervention found to be effective in one site might be effective in another:

It would be naïve to believe that the quality of evidence to guide practice in health promotion was such that decisions concerning methods and organisation will ever be routine. The complexity of the factors which influence individual behaviours, exposure to risk, and the capacity of individuals and communities to change their circumstances mean that research evidence will always need to be adapted to fit local circumstances.

(Nutbeam 1996)

Whether interventions are feasible, achieve coverage and are acceptable

An intervention that can be delivered feasibly by its providers, can actually reach those potential recipients it targets and is regarded as acceptable by those who receive it in one site, may not be so in another. If any one of these factors is not achieved, the intervention is unlikely to be effective in a new site.

An intervention that is not fully delivered will obviously not achieve optimal effects, and the feasibility of delivery will depend on context. For example, providers will vary in their managerial ability and capacity to implement an intervention (Nutbeam 1996). This might in turn be influenced by: the presence of a supportive policy environment or suitable institutional home for the intervention; the presence of an influential 'champion' for the intervention within the provider agency; or the willingness of local stakeholders to participate actively in the delivery of an intervention that requires this. For example, the recruitment and deployment of peer educators might prove feasible in one site but not in others. The feasibility of some interventions will require the presence of other services. For example, an intervention supporting couples to check whether they have concordant HIV statuses before engaging in unprotected sex would require the presence of HIV voluntary counselling and testing services.

In order to achieve its potential, an intervention also needs to reach the target population. The extent to which a population can access an intervention might, for example, depend on their access to general health services if the intervention is delivered via these, or the ability of providers to reach out to a population in other ways.

An intervention must not only reach its targets but also be regarded as acceptable by them if it is to stand any chance of having an impact. A population must find an intervention acceptable enough to get or stay involved with, or to pay attention to its message. Judgements by populations of intervention acceptability will depend on prevailing social norms. There is some evidence, for example, that condom promotion has proved acceptable and subsequently effective in urban, but not rural, Tanzania (Munguti et al. 1997), and in Thai, but not Indian, brothels (Grosskurth and Kumaranayake 2003). Similarly, HIV prevention peer education for gay men appears to have been acceptable when delivered in US bars (Kelly et al. 1992) but not in UK gyms (Hart and Elford 2003). Acceptability may have economic dimensions. For example, HIV voluntary counselling and testing services that require clients to attend clinics twice (first to be tested and then to receive results) may be unacceptable to some populations because of the transport and opportunity costs involved (Grosskurth and Kumaranayake 2003).

Activity 16.1

An intervention to educate gay men about the important role of condoms in preventing HIV transmission in 'casual' sex was found to have a significant impact on the incidence of HIV in small American towns in a 1992 study. If you were considering whether to implement the intervention in a small UK town, what factors do you think would affect whether the intervention is feasible, achieves adequate coverage and is acceptable in the new site?

 Feedback

Whether the intervention will be feasible might be affected by whether a local agency to do the work actually exists; whether there are any gay bars in the town; whether these will allow the intervention to occur on their premises; and whether peer educators can be recruited among local gay men. Coverage might be affected by whether local gay men who are at risk of HIV transmission use the bars and whether the peer educators can make contact and undertake interventions with these men. Acceptability might be affected by whether local gay men are comfortable discussing sex and HIV infection while they are out socializing in the bars and whether the peer educators are judged as appropriate sources of information by these men.

Whether interventions address key population needs

A further factor that determines the potential transferability of intervention effectiveness is how the intended aims of the intervention relate to the needs of the population in the new site.

The rates of disease in a population are influenced by certain 'risk' behaviours. In the case of HIV, for example, such behaviours might include: early age of sexual debut; high frequency of sexual partners; large degree of concurrence of sexual relationships; and low use of condoms. Risk behaviours are in turn influenced by a range of psychosocial factors. Regarding HIV, these could range from individuals' lack of knowledge, ability and autonomy to negotiate sex etc. to the overall status of women or patterns of migration of particular sub-groups within the population. If the psychosocial factors that influence behaviour can ethically and practically be influenced by health promotion interventions then they can be regarded as constituting 'needs'.

Health promotion interventions aim to influence the incidence of diseases or other outcomes by changing behaviours as a result of addressing psychosocial needs. An intervention might have exactly the same effect on a psychosocial factor in two sites but have completely different knock-on effects on behaviours and disease rates within each site. For example, an intervention that increases sexual health knowledge is more likely to influence behaviour when lack of such knowledge is the key psychosocial factor limiting individuals' potential for behaviour change, i.e. when knowledge is a key need. When another psychosocial factor, such as power to exercise any control over sex, is the key need, an intervention addressing knowledge alone is unlikely to be effective (Grosskurth and Kumaranayake 2003). In such a site, an intervention to address knowledge might be effective only if accompanied by an intervention to address empowerment. Thus, the sites to which the intervention is likely to be most transferable will be determined by the match between the aims of the intervention and the needs present within particular populations. This in turn will be influenced by the presence and effects of other interventions being deployed within that site.

What is true of the relationship between psychosocial factors and behaviours is also true of the relationship between behaviours and diseases. For example, an intervention that reduces unprotected sex among sex workers is likely to have a bigger overall impact on HIV incidence within an 'immature' HIV epidemic when relatively more transmissions occur within such 'high risk' groups than in a mature one where a greater proportion of infections will be occurring in the 'general' population. This implies that the psychosocial factors influencing the key behaviours influencing disease rates will constitute more important needs than those driving other behaviours. Thus, the transferability of the effectiveness of an intervention is influenced by the epidemiology of the disease in question in a particular site.

In other words, different populations/sites will have different psychosocial 'needs'. Needs should therefore be assessed prior to the implementation of health promotion interventions, to ensure that the aims of the interventions that come to be delivered in the site correspond to the most important determinants of disease in that population.

What has been described above is analogous to 'interventions' aiming to promote growth of ailing plants. A plant's growth requires light, water and minerals. These are potential limiting factors on plant growth and constitute 'needs' if they are absent. Watering the plant will be an 'effective intervention' for plants whose lack of growth results from lack of water. This intervention's effectiveness will not however transfer to plants whose lack of growth results from a need for light, which requires another intervention such as provision of sunlight.

 Activity 16.2

Remember the intervention described in the last activity. If, this time, you were considering whether to implement the intervention in the same American towns today, what epidemiological and psychosocial factors do you think might influence whether the intervention achieved the same impact as it did in 1992? You should assume the intervention will be feasible, achieve good coverage, be acceptable to gay men and will improve knowledge among men who lack this.

 Feedback

Whether the intervention actually had an impact on rates of HIV would be influenced by: whether HIV infections among gay men accounted for a significant proportion of infections in the town; what proportion of HIV transmissions among gay men occurred between casual rather than long-term partners; how extensive was lack of knowledge among men; and whether there are other important factors influencing risk such as non-consensual sex, condoms breaking or slipping off, men assuming that their partners are the same HIV status as themselves, or men choosing not to prioritize avoidance of HIV infection.

Evidence-informed intervention transfer

Providers who are considering adopting an intervention ideally require a detailed assessment of: its original process of planning, delivery and receipt; evaluation of the contextual factors which promoted or impeded feasibility; coverage and acceptability in the original site; and the intervention's aims and how these corresponded to the needs of the evaluation study population and to those of the population of concern to the new provider. This information will allow providers to decide: whether to adopt the intervention; if so, how to modify it to maximize performance; and whether other interventions should be provided to maximize the meeting of the key needs of the new population.

Unfortunately, evaluations of interventions published in scientific journals rarely report how interventions were planned, delivered and received, how these processes were influenced by the context (Nutbeam 1996; Kegeles *et al.* 2000), what modifications might be indicated to maximize feasibility, accessibility and acceptability of the intervention in other sites or how intervention aims matched population needs. Such information can sometimes be obtained via evaluators' websites or by contacting the evaluators or intervention providers to obtain intervention documentation, manuals and training materials, or to discuss the intervention. Evaluators (and those funding evaluations) should consider the potential transferability of interventions as an integral part of evaluation and report this as part of the dissemination of their findings.

The US Center for Disease Control (CDC) has sponsored a programme of HIV prevention intervention transfer in which the evaluators of interventions demonstrated as effective then work with new adopters to modify and implement these in new sites (Kegeles *et al.* 2000; Spink Neumann and Sogolow 2000). Interventions such as peer education, community development and one-to-one counselling have been successfully transferred. Certain aspects of interventions are treated as core components, either on the basis of evidence or (more often) opinion that these are required for intervention effectiveness. Some aspects of interventions, such as education sessions, are required to be replicated in standard format while other aspects, especially those involving community development activities, can be more freely modified to suit local circumstances as long as they continue to be informed by the underlying theory and hypothesized mechanism of action of the original intervention (Kegeles *et al.* 2000). For example, one community development project for young gay men emphasized the importance of organizing 'fun' events in its hypothesized mechanism of action. What was regarded as 'fun', however, in the new Texan intervention sites (e.g. football games) was very different to that in the original Californian sites (Kegeles *et al.* 2000).

The CDC programme identified that intervention guidance worked best when: written guidance was supplemented with face-to-face support and videos; frequent use was made of examples; care was taken to ensure wording was neither patronizing, over-complex nor offensive; recommendations directed a specific course of action including a proper explanation of the rationale for this; images used were demographically inclusive; and advice on which groups an intervention might target was provided. Intervention modification was viewed both as a means to maximize the fit between an intervention and its new context, as well as to promote ownership of the intervention by its new adopters (Kegeles *et al.* 2000). Finally, those involved in the programme suggested that a role existed for 'transfer agents' who would mediate between evaluators and providers, supporting the process of intervention modification and transfer, but such work has not been evaluated to date.

It may be important for interventions transferred from one site or population to another to be empirically re-evaluated. Whereas in the original evaluation, the key question is likely to have been whether and under what conditions the intervention was effective, the aim of the re-evaluation may instead be to assess whether the intervention can feasibly and acceptably be delivered in a new site to a new population (Nutbeam 1996).

Scaling up interventions

Scale-up is one particular, but very important, example of intervention transfer in which interventions previously provided within the context of pilots are transferred to a wider set of sites and populations. In line with what was stated earlier, most health promoters are likely to prefer to see the full-scale deployment of interventions that have already been piloted and found to be effective, and most evaluators would hope that the interventions they subject to evaluation, if found to be effective, would be scaled up so that they benefit as many people as possible.

Scale-up can bring about 'added value' in terms of impact. When a health promotion intervention reaches and influences a critical mass of individuals directly, it is often more likely to produce indirect, multiplicative effects whereby the attitudes, behaviours or states of disease of individuals brought about by the intervention then start to influence these states in other individuals. This can be particularly the case with interventions addressing infectious diseases, where an individual's risk of infection is influenced by the behaviours and prevalence of infection among those around them. It is also the case where interventions influence social norms about risk behaviours. Scale-up can also bring about greater efficiency through economies of scale so that financial inputs per outcome achieved are reduced. However, the process of scaling up interventions from pilot evaluations to larger-scale implementation is not straightforward. This section considers the issues that should be considered in order to maximize the likely effectiveness of scaled-up interventions.

Intervention fidelity and modification

As discussed above, intervention effectiveness depends on epidemiological and psychosocial context, and therefore delivery involving unmodified replication of the intervention across different populations would in many cases produce sub-optimal impact. Scale-up can instead proceed via each population receiving a form of the intervention where, although the intervention retains its core elements, the aims and objectives are adapted towards the specific behaviours and psychosocial factors driving disease in each population, i.e. to their specific health promotion needs. Interventions can also be allowed to vary slightly, in a planned manner, in order that they are maximally feasible, achieving coverage and acceptable in each new site.

Provider capacity

Scaled-up interventions differ from pilot interventions in a number of ways that require consideration in order to maximize feasibility of delivery. Scaled-up interventions involve more staff and therefore require more management capacity. Staff involved in 'routine' delivery within scale-ups may be less personally committed to making interventions work than those involved in 'innovative' pilot work, especially when the latter were closely involved in designing the intervention and therefore feel 'ownership' of it. Evaluations of scale-ups from the USA suggest staff are more likely to feel motivated to deliver an intervention if they are first engaged in a discussion about the processes and outcomes of the original intervention, and participate in decisions about how the work should be taken forward in the scale-up (Rotherham-Borus *et al.* 2000), as is the case in the CDC work discussed earlier (Kegeles *et al.* 2000; Spink Neumann and Sogolow 2000).

A pilot intervention will generally be regarded as a specific project that is necessarily an add-on to the work of the agency involved. However, this can no longer be the case when an intervention is scaled up. If it is to be sustainable and properly supported and managed over the long term, the planning and delivery of a scaled-up intervention must be 'institutionalized' within the agency or agencies providing it. This might, for example, involve the intervention being linked into the agency's overall mission and objectives, the administration of the intervention being performed by general rather than project-specific staff, and intervention staff and managers being directly accountable to the general managers of the agency and subject to standard policies and procedures, and terms and conditions.

Inter-agency collaboration

As well as the challenges introduced by the involvement of large numbers of new staff, scale-up generally also usually involves more complex arrays of provider organizations and other stakeholders. This occurs both because the intervention is being delivered across broader areas but also because whereas pilot studies are often based in a single agency, often located in a research institution, scaled-up interventions more often will involve ongoing contributions of specialists working in different agencies. The sustainability of implementation of scale-up services will also generally depend on the cooperation and goodwill of an even broader range of 'stakeholders', these being defined as those whose support is necessary to make the intervention work.

Whereas all aspects of delivery are usually within the control of a single manager in a pilot study, scale-up usually requires multiple managers from different agencies to coordinate their actions. Processes of cooperation and communication between the various providers and stakeholders can be informed by stakeholder analysis exercises in which each party's needs are assessed and understood (Varvasovsky and Brugha 2000). It has been suggested on the basis of evaluations of integrated rural development projects that where scaled-up work involves different sectors, the coordination of these cannot be expected to occur purely at a national level and instead requires local inter-sectoral cooperation (Binswanger 2000).

Quality control and evaluation

Monitoring is important to ensure that a scaled-up intervention is delivered as intended, either faithfully to the original intervention or modified in a planned manner. With rapid upscaling there is the risk that mistakes and problems rapidly become amplified and therefore more difficult to solve (Grosskurth and Kumaranayake 2003). There is evidence from failures in the scale-up of integrated rural development projects in the 1970s and 1980s that there is greater potential for error in the scale-up of complex compared with simple interventions (Binswanger 2000). To minimize the potential for 'error amplification', scale-up should occur step-wise, for example by geographical area or sector, and each phase should involve adequate piloting and monitoring.

Financial management

Financial management of scale-up can also involve particular challenges. Scale-up is likely to require programmes to secure local or mainstream resources and be less reliant on external or developmental funding if the work is to be sustainable. Whereas pilots are often generously supported by research funders, scaled up, 'routine' services may be less well supported. Providers must determine whether a scaled-up intervention is actually financially viable and what implications any cost reductions that are deemed necessary will have for intervention feasibility and effectiveness (Rotherham-Borus *et al.* 2000). The need for cost reductions may be offset by the fact that scale-up can bring about decreases in unit costs because of economies of scale. There may be points during the expansion however when the increased volume of activity requires a specific increase in infrastructure, equipment or staffing, necessitating a 'step-change' in investment.

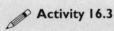 **Activity 16.3**

An HIV prevention intervention planned and delivered by a university research unit aiming to distribute condoms to adolescents and educate them about HIV was delivered in eight refugee camps in one region of Sudan. It was found to be effective in reducing HIV transmission. Think about what sorts of organizational and logistic decisions might need to be made if the intervention was to be scaled up to all refugee camps across Sudan.

Feedback

Issues about which decisions would need to be made would include the following: whether the intervention should be modified to meet the needs and cultural expectations of different populations in each camp; whether another organization or organizations should take on the implementation of the intervention; whether all aspects of the intervention should be delivered by a single agency working in each region or whether different agencies should lead on different aspects of the interventions across the whole country; what role if any might the research unit play; how new staff in the provider agencies would be trained and supervised; how the whole programme would be led; how the different organizations involved would liaise with one another; how the agencies managing the refugee camps and the other agencies providing services in the refugee camps would be involved in the programme; whether and how the various populations using the refugee camps should be involved; how condoms, educational materials and staff would be transported over the much larger areas involved in the scale-up; whether each collaborating agency should be responsible for monitoring and quality or whether a single agency should lead on this; whether the scale-up should be evaluated and if so in order to answer what questions; how the scale-up will be financed; and what financial management procedures are required.

Summary

Interventions found to be effective in one site cannot be assumed to have exactly the same effects in another. This is so not only because of inter-site differences in the contextual factors that promote and impede the feasibility, coverage and acceptability of interventions, but also because of differences in the needs that must be addressed in order to prevent disease or promote health in different populations. Interventions should be modified as necessary to maximize their potential effectiveness when implemented in other sites, if possible informed by an assessment of detailed information on: the planning, delivery and uptake of the original intervention; how original delivery and receipt was influenced by context: how intervention aims related to the needs of the evaluation study population and relate to the needs of the populations to which the intervention is to be transferred. Scale-up represents a particularly important example of intervention transfer whereby interventions move from piloting with a relatively small number of participants to much larger-scale delivery. This can bring added value in terms of impact as well as economies of scale. However, scale-up presents new challenges in areas such as intervention modification, provider capacity, inter-agency collaboration, quality control and financial management.

References

Binswanger HP (2000) Scaling up HIV/AIDS programs to national coverage. *Science*, 288: 2173–6.

Grosskurth H, Kumaranayake L (2003) Generalizability of trials and implementation of research into practice, in J Stephenson, J Imrie, C. Bonell (eds) *Effective Sexual Health Interventions: Issues in experimental evaluation*. Oxford: Oxford University Press.

Hart G, Elford J (2003) The limits of generalizability: community-based sexual health interventions among gay men, in J Stephenson, J Imrie, C. Bonell (eds) *Effective Sexual Health Interventions: Issues in experimental evaluation*. Oxford: Oxford University Press.

Kegeles SM, Rebchook GM, Hays RB, Terry MA, O'Donnell L, Leonard NR, Kelly JA, Spink Neumann M (2000) From science to application: the development of an intervention package. *AIDS Education and Prevention*, 12(Supplement A): 62–74.

Kelly JA, St Lawrence JA, Stevenson LY, Hauth AC, Kalichman SC, Diaz YE, Brasfield TL, Koob JJ, Morgan M (1992) Community AIDS/HIV risk reduction: the effects of endorsements by popular people in three cities. *American Journal of Public Health*, **82**(11): 1483–9.

Munguti K, Grosskurth H, Newell J, Senkoro K, Mosha F, Todd J, Mayaud P, Gavyole A, Quigley M, Hayes R (1997) Patterns of sexual behaviour in a rurual population in north-western Tanzania. *Social Science & Medicine*, 44: 1553–661.

Nutbeam D (1996) Improving the fit between research and practice in health promotion: overcoming structural barriers. *Canadian Journal of Public Health*, 87(6, Supplement 2): 18–22.

Rotherham-Borus MJ, Rebchook GM, Kelly JA, Adams J, Spink Neumann M (2000) Bridging research and practice: community-researcher partnerships for replicating effective interventions. *AIDS Education and Prevention*, 12(Supplement A).

Spink Neumann M, Sogolow E (2000) Replicating effective programs: HIV/AIDS prevention technology transfer. *AIDS Education and Prevention*, 12(Supplement A): 35–48.

Varvasovsky Z, Brugha R (2000) How to do a stakeholder analysis. *Health Policy and Planning*, 15(3): 338–45.

Glossary

Acceptability Whether an intervention is acceptable to the recipients of or those providing an intervention.

Agenda-setting Process by which the media influence what the public and policy makers perceive to be important.

Aim An expanded and refined version of a goal that sets out the means by which the end point, in general terms, is to be attained.

Ambivalence A conflict between two courses of action each of which has perceived costs and benefits associated with it. The exploration and resolution of ambivalence is a key feature in motivational interviewing.

Background noise Influences on the target audience other than the intervention, which make it difficult to attribute outcomes to the intervention.

Behavioural Observable, quantifiable pattern of human behaviour.

Change talk Involves a client expressing personal advantages of changing behaviour, optimism for change, intention to change and the disadvantages of no change or the status quo.

Cognitive Thought processes such as attention, concentration, perception, thinking, learning, memory, beliefs, expectations and assumptions.

Community A neighbourhood and/or group with common interests and identity.

Community asset mapping An inventory of the strengths (assets) of the people who make up a community; the interconnections of these assets and how to access them.

Community development The process of change in neighbourhoods and communities. It aims to increase the extent and effectiveness of community action, community activity and agencies' relationships with communities.

Competitive analysis Assessments of what competing organizations (such as the tobacco companies) are doing in order to inform efforts to control or compensate for these.

Consumer orientation Why people choose to do as they do – what ideas, emotions and aspirations influence them.

Coverage The extent to which an intervention is received by those it targets.

Creative epidemiology Presenting statistics in ways that make them more meaningful to the media and the public.

Critical appraisal The consistent assessment of research studies in order to determine the validity or trustworthiness of the evidence they contain.

Customer defined quality What the user thinks of an intervention or service.

Diffusion acceleration The rapidity with which messages may be disseminated, once the process of transmission from one, to two or more agencies has begun.

Edutainment Learning through media, particularly mass media, that both educates and entertains.

Effectiveness The extent to which an intervention produces a beneficial result under usual circumstances.

Empowerment Individuals are given knowledge, skills and opportunity to develop a sense of control and mastery over life circumstances.

Evaluation The critical assessment of the value of an activity.

Feasibility A characteristic of issues for which there is a practical solution.

Fidelity The extent to which a subsequent implementation of an intervention is faithful in terms of the process of delivery to how the intervention was implemented in the original site.

Formative evaluation An evaluation aiming to refine the process by which an intervention is delivered.

Framing How an issue is presented in the media.

Free-text terms Inconsistently applied terms taken from the text of a reference, used to catalogue research studies.

Health equity auditing Identifies how fairly services or other resources are distributed in relation to the health needs of different groups and areas, and the priority action to provide services.

Health impact assessment An approach to ensure that decision-making at all levels considers the potential impacts of decisions on health and health inequalities, and identifies actions that can enhance positive effects and reduce or eliminate negative effects.

Health inequalities Differences in health experience and health status between countries, regions and socioeconomic groups.

Health needs assessment A systematic process of identifying priority health issues, targeting the populations with most need and taking action in the most cost effective and efficient way.

Health-related behaviour Things people do that affect their health (e.g. sexual activity that involves exposure to infections).

Health-related needs Attributes people need to have to be able to control their health-related behaviour: knowledge and awareness; access to resources; interpersonal skills and physical motor skills; and bodily autonomy.

Indexing (thesaurus) terms Consistently applied database-specific terms used to catalogue research studies.

Intervention A purposeful activity using finite resources that occurs in a specific place with the aim of changing something specific for a specific person or group of people.

Mass media Electronic and print channels through which information is transmitted to a large number of people at a time.

Media advocacy The strategic use of mass media as a resource for advancing a social or public policy initiative.

Modification A planned process of altering an intervention to ensure it maximally addresses health promotion needs and is feasible, achieves adequate coverage and is acceptable in a new site of implementation.

Motivation Incentives or driving forces that encourage the adoption of health-promoting behaviours or lifestyles.

Motivational interviewing A client-centred, directive method for enhancing intrinsic motivation to change by exploring and resolving ambivalence.

Multiplier effect The additional impact achieved when an intervention uses several agencies to pass on a message, each of which convey the message to several other agencies and so on.

Normative need The capacity for a population to benefit from a health promotion intervention.

Objective Concrete and specific elaboration of an aim.

Outcome evaluation Research that determines the end results of an intervention.

Outcomes measures Change in status as a result of the system processes (in the health services context, the change in health status as a result of care).

Participation A process through which stakeholders influence and share control over development initiatives and the decisions and resources which affect them.

Peer education The teaching or sharing of information, values and behaviours between individuals with shared characteristics such as behaviour, experience, status or social and cultural backgrounds.

Pilot An initial, small-scale implementation of an intervention accompanied by an evaluation of its process and/or outcomes.

Plan A time-limited document describing programmes, strategies and projects and how they relate to each other

Process The use of resources or the activity within a system.

Process evaluation Evaluation that concentrates on examining the process of an intervention.

Programme A collection of interventions that share an overall health-related goal.

Readiness Used in motivational interviewing to refer to the degree to which a client is resolved to change their lifestyle or behaviour.

Relapse prevention A technique whereby people become aware of the antecedents of their own risk-related behaviour and learn to implement behavioural strategies that are incompatible with the risk behaviour but still achieve the same function in reducing stress and tension.

Relationship marketing Action to build ongoing, mutually beneficial relationships with target groups.

Resistance Opposition to changing behaviour, often expressed as a series of 'excuses' for not wanting or needing to change.

Scale-up The implementation of an intervention previously provided in the context of a pilot across a wider area and/or to a broader population.

Search filter A combination of index and free-text terms designed to search a database in order to locate every possible and yet relevant research study.

Setting (site) The place or location in which intervention activities occur.

Settings for health The place or social context in which people engage in daily activities in which environmental, organizational and personal factors interact to affect health and well-being.

Social determinants of health Conditions which affect people's health such as their working and living environments, income, social networks and social position.

Social learning theory A theory suggesting that individuals learn and then change their behaviour by observing and then modelling the behaviour of others.

Stakeholder marketing Activities aiming to influence the behaviour of those groups who shape the social environment (e.g. policy-makers or health professionals).

Strategy A plan informed by evidence, values and theories that sets global and specific aims and describes how these will be achieved.

Summative evaluation An evaluation aiming to establish the value of an intervention.

Sustainability The extent to which an intervention may be continued beyond its initial implementation; this may be dependent upon a continued source of funding, programme effectiveness or changing priorities.

Systematic review A review of the literature that uses an explicit approach to searching, selecting and combining the relevant studies.

Theatre for development Community theatre used both for action research and as a verification tool in development programmes.

Theatre in education An umbrella term describing the use of scripted, live theatre usually linked to an interactive workshop used to explore a range of social issues and meet educational aims.

Theatre in health education Uses the techniques of theatre in education in the service of health education.

Theatre of the oppressed A form of popular theatre of, by and for those engaged in the struggle for liberation. The starting point is not an explicit educational objective, but rather individual and social development and empowerment.

Transferability The extent to which the results of a study as it applies to a particular patient group or setting hold true for another population or context.

Transtheoretical model Developed to describe and explain the different stages in behaviour change. The model is based on the premise that behaviour change is a process, not an event, and that individuals have different levels of motivation or readiness to change.

Views study Research that asks and reports on people's perspectives, opinions, beliefs or attitudes about a topic of interest (such as a particular intervention or social exclusion).

Index

Page numbers for figures have suffix **f**, those for tables have suffix **t**